HEART ATTACK!!!: WHAT NOW?

Heart Attack!!!: What Now?

It's NOT Cholesterol!

A review of findings on cardiac disease with guidelines for effective treatment and prevention with particular emphasis on outdated methods

WHAT EVERY DOCTOR AND PATIENT NEEDS TO KNOW

Dr Willem Serfontein

Library of Congress Control Number: 2011900480
ISBN: Hardcover   978-1-4568-5071-5
                         Softcover   978-1-4568-5070-8
                         Ebook   978-1-4568-5072-2

Cover design: J Pienaar

This book was created in the United States of America.

To order additional copies of this book, contact:
Xlibris Corporation
0-800-644-6988
www.xlibrispublishing.co.uk
Orders@xlibrispublishing.co.uk
300886

CONTENTS

DISCLAIMER

This book is not a prescription for the treatment and prevention of heart disease. It offers important information from the relevant literature aimed at enabling both doctor and patient to select the best approach for each patient. Ultimately the patient—preferably in consultation with his/her doctor—should choose which treatment will be the most beneficial in his/her case.

Due to the number of variables arising from the treatment of cardiac disease, and the differing individual responses to treatment, it is impossible to guarantee success. I am not a clinician. My purpose as a medical scientist is to evaluate the latest findings and to present these to both doctor and patient for consideration.

The many viewpoints presented by the different authors quoted in the referencesare, by their very nature, their own, and not necessarily mine.

I strongly urge patients not to apply their own methods of treatment, but rather to design their treatment programmes in full collaboration with their doctors, who understand the latest developments in medicine. It is also important that the patient should grasp the relevant principles in order to be self motivated, without which the chances of a successful outcome are greatly reduced.

FURTHER STUDY

The volume of information that has been published on coronary heart disease is so vast that is is impossible to do justice to the topic in a single publication such as this. It is therefore vital that the patient should read as widely as possible on the topic. Below is a list of some of the more significant publications as recommended reading.

1. Lundell, D: *The Great Cholesterol Lie*, ISBN #9780979034015.
2. Peskin, B S, and Habib A: T*he Hidden Story of Cancer*, Pinnacle Press, Houston, USA, p 277
3. Lundell, D. 2010. T*he Great Statin Scam*. Total Health Breakthroughs
4. *Statins and Cancer Risk*, Townsend Letter, FebMarch, 2008, p55
5. "Composition of Plaque": *Lancet* 1994, 344: 1195.
6. "Lowering LDL does not prevent heart attacks", *J Am Phys Surg* 2005, 10: 83
7. "Low cholesterol does not prevent heart disease", *JAMA*, 1994, 272: 1335
8. The Vytorin Trial: *JAMA* 2007, 297: 1344
9. Cholesterol Drugs: The danger. *Health Intelligence*, 2010 Edn 2, p 48
10. lSerfontein, W.J. 2001. *New Nutrition*. Cape Town: Tafelberg.

THE OLD AND NEW APPROACHES TO HEART DISEASE

The level of thinking that caused the problem cannot be used to solve the problem—Albert Einstein

I am in possession of a pamphlet compiled and distributed by a large pharmaceutical company ("Big Pharma") with the stated purpose of informing the public about cholesterol and the role it plays in heart disease. Clearly, the intention of the pamphlet is to promote the company's products, including statins, which lower cholesterol. If one could believe everything in the pamphlet literally, there would be no option but to conclude that the pharmaceutical companies are in possession of the solution to heart problems; all that is needed is for everyone, including doctors, to believe and comply with what the pamphlet says, although no supporting scientific findings are given.

We should remember that the public has been following the prescriptive guidelines contained in this pamphlet for over 20 years at the insistence of the medical profession, and yet the death toll from heart attacks is steadily increasing.

The problem is that none of the fundamental statements made in the pamphlet is true, and they are being increasing questioned and contradicted by new information. The entire pamphlet is therefore meaningless, outdated and completely misleading.

For this reason I have decided to consolidate the relevant information and to present it in this book for the use of all who are involved, especially medical doctors and cardiac patients.

HISTORICAL SURVEY

Coronary heart disease is an example of a condition which has only in the last 70 years become a serious medical problem. Despite billions of dollars spent on research, medical science has no solution. Considerable attention has been given to cholesterol as its possible cause, but as more information becomes available, this turns out to be the less true.

The disease is characterised by the accretion of a fatty deposit (plaque) on the inside of the veins in certain sections of the vascular system. It includes relatively small quantities of cholesterol, but also many other components including calcium. Additionally, the cholesterol is not present as free cholesterol (as is often stated), but instead as *cholesterolesters* of which some are in an oxidised form. Cholesterol is a fatty substance which is produced in the liver as required. It plays an essential precursor role in the synthesis of steroid hormones and bile acids; a cholesterol deficiency may even be the cause of reduced hormone levels. This is the conclusion reached by a recent study by Dzugan and Smith (*Life Extension,* Feb. 2003, p1).

The suppression of cholesterol synthesis in the body could therefore have serious clinical consequences.

When the arteries, particularly the coronary arteries, are so constricted by the accretion of plaque (or by a blood clot) that the supply of blood and thus the function of the heart is jeopardised, a heart attack ensues. It was previously accepted, without real evidence, that saturated fats such as butter were the cause of raised blood cholesterol levels and thus the cause of heart attacks. Many researchers no longer accept this.

Heart attacks as we know them today were very rare before 1920. Between 1920 and 1990 the frequency rose rapidly (19301960), followed by a decline in certain countries (19601990). There is no evidence that medical intervention was responsible for either the escalations or reductions.

By 1900, coronary heart disease was not entirely unknown as a scientific phenomenon. It had been described in medical text books even earlier. However, its occurrence was very scarce in the first quarter of the twentieth century; it was virtually unknown before 1926.

Two British doctors, Finlayson and Mackinnon, independently compiled data on the frequency of the disease in two separate British regions. D.R. Finlayson worked in the London area and recorded deaths due to cardiac failure since 1868 from hospital records (*J Roy Coll Gen Pract*, April 1987, 174). He expressed the results as the relative occurrence of the illness per 1000 members of the population over a given period. The following table illustrates his findings:

Period	Relative occurrence of deaths from heart disease
1869 1900	
1900—1910	10
1900 1980	80

As the figures indicate, from 1869 to 1900 the illness was very scarce; also, it did not increase in frequency during this period. A sharp rise in deaths from heart disease was recorded between 1900 and 1910; in 1910 there were ten times as many deaths per 1000 members of the society surveyed than in 1900. Nevertheless, the occurrence of the disease was still very negligible even in comparison to 1926 when deaths from heart disease were still regarded as rare. (*New Engl J Med* 2002, 347: 81).

After 1926, heart deaths rose rapidly; by 1980 there were 80 times as many such deaths per 1000 of the population than in 1900.

These findings were confirmed by Dr. A. Mackinnon, working independently in a different region (Yorkshire) (*ibid*). This survey was performed in a rural area on a population of 22 000 and confirmed both the tenfold increase in the years 1900 to 1910 and the 80fold increase between 1900 and1980.

It was and still is not clear what caused this sudden rise in heart deaths. Both authors believed the increase in the periodb19001910 resulted from mass produced cigarettes which had come on to the market at that stage, and the fact that 80% of men had begun to smoke these cigarettes. Neither of the authors could offer an explanation for the 80fold increase by 1980.

Today the effects of smoking remain undisputed, but it is also accepted that other causes exist and that smoking is but one of our health problems; probably not even the most important.

Other salient causes have arisen since 1926, most likely associated with industrialisation, urbanisation and the consequent variations in food source, lifestyle and diet changes, including a considerable increase in refined carbohydrates. Another significant problem, which is only now being realised, is the role chronic inflammatory conditions play in heart disease.

HOW DOES A HEART ATTACK COME ABOUT?

The heart is made up of, inter alia, muscles and a vascular system which pumps bloodto the heart muscle and through the body at a contraction tempo of about 72 per minute. In this process, oxygen and nutritients reach the heart muscle via the coronary vessels, without which it cannot function. There are 3 main coronary vessels: the left anterior (front) descending heart vessel (LAD), the circumflex, and the right coronary vessels, each of which serves a specific area of the heart.

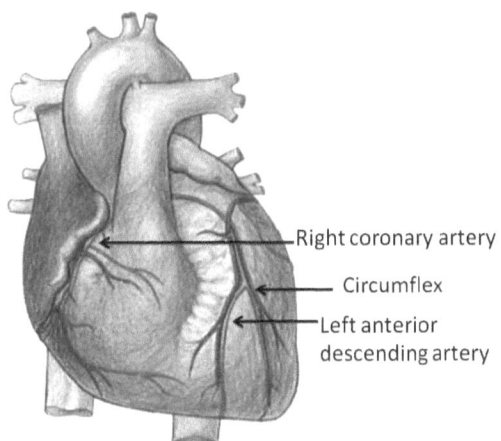

Right coronary artery

Circumflex

Left anterior descending artery

Fig 1

The coronary arteries contain muscle fibres in their walls. By way of alternating contraction and relaxation of the heart muscles, the heart pumps blood to the various sections of the heart as well as to various anatomical areas of the body.

Coronary spasm occurs when these muscles contract spastically, just as various other muscles of the body may go into spasm, which in

some cases is caused by deficiencies in the supply of certain minerals (magnesium, calcium) to these muscles.

The typical discomfort of a coronary spasm often develops in the resting state—usually in the early morning hours. When the spasm is relieved (spontaneously or assisted by medication), the heart returns to its normal mode of function. The temporary shortage of blood supply to the heart muscle results in a feeling of discomfort in the chest, which is so typical of this condition. Prolonged heart muscle spasm can, however, result in permanent damage to the heart muscle, or even a heart attack.

Atherosclerosis is the commonest cause of blockages to coronary blood supply. This results in a more permanent reduction of blood flow to the heart muscle. The accompanying figures demonstrate both the appearance of the inner surface of a healthy coronary vessel and the appearance of one with signs of atherosclerosis.

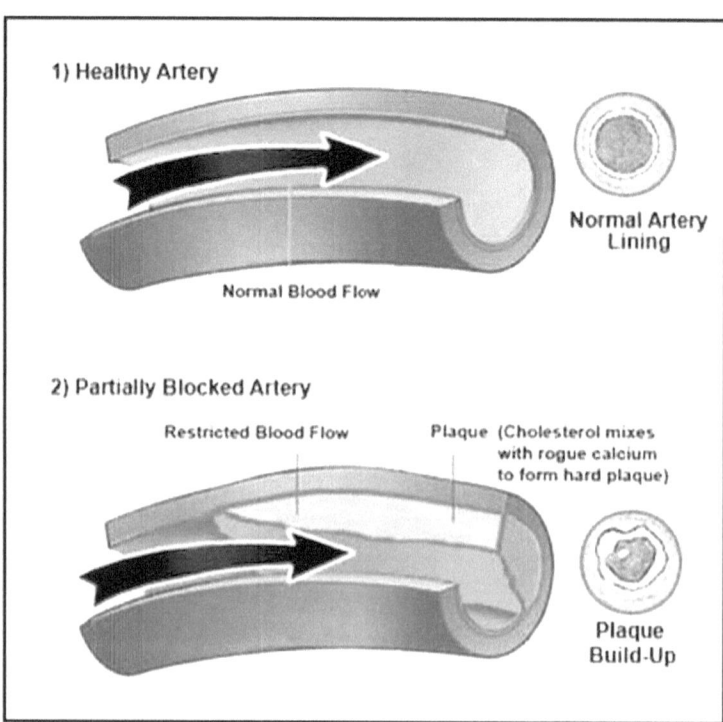

Fig. 2

As we grow older, deposits start to form on the inner surface of the artery walls. These deposits are refered to as "plaque".

The process of atherosclerosis can be summarised as follows:

- Cholesterol in the body (e.g. blood, artery walls) is present, not as free cholesterol, but mostly as esters of cholesterol (e.g. in LDL) with certain long chain fatty acids, e.g. linoleic acid.
- When oxidation of cholesterol occurs (as may happen in the industrial processing of foodstuffs, e.g. sunflower oil) such oxidation is found mainly in the side chains of the cholesterol esters, as abnormal cholesterol derivatives are formed (more about this below).
- These abnormal LDL then enter the artery wall.
- This causes inflammatory cytokines to be released. These attract white blood cells or monocytes to this area of the artery wall.
- The monocytes proceed to absorb the abnormal LDL, overloading the white blood cells with cholesterol esters.
- This causes them to take on a "foamy" appearance (called foam cells).
- As the foam cells join together, visible "fatty streaks" appear in the arterial wall.
- In an effort to heal the damage, smooth muscle cells migrate from the surrounding media area of the arterial wall.
- This causes the damaged area (plaque) to expand, and ultimately it develops a fibrous cap over the fatty streaks.
- In combination with each other, these deposits give rise to inflammatory changes, which later cause the fibrous cap to weaken, and even to rupture.
- The result may lead to the formation of a blood clot.

The ultimate result of a blood clot brought about by clotting in an artery which has become constricted by plaque is a heart attack. It may have its origin in local clot formation in the heart, but such a blood clot may also be transported to the heart by the blood stream from elsewhere in the body, e.g. in the lungs.

In both cases the flow of blood to that area of the heart muscle that is served by a particular artery may become severely blocked.

Plaque that forms locally can be one of two types. The one type is known as "unstable plaque". If such unstable plaque ruptures, it can result in a localised blood clot.

Stable plaque, on the other hand, does not rupture readily, but as it builds up it may progressively block the artery to such an extent that the flow of blood to the heart muscle is seriously compromised.

WHAT CONSTITUTES PLAQUE?

The earlier theory, that heart attacks are caused by cholesterol and saturated fats, postulated that plaque consists mainly of cholesterol deposits in the artery walls, together with saturated fats and substances such as calcium and certain other cells, besides triglyceride fats and cellular metabolic products.

However, more recent investigations into the composition of plaque have revealed that this is only partly true. A fairly recent article in *Lancet* has shown that plaque contains more than 10 different molecular components, but no saturated fats (*Lancet* 1994, 344:1195). Cholesterol is indeed a component of plaque, but not in quantities that could cause the blockage of arteries. According to these findings, any cholesterol that is present in plaque is in response to tissue damage, as happens in all other instances of tissue damage, and it constitutes an element of the healing process.

Other studies regarding the composition of plaque came to more or less the same conclusion.

So the original question remained: What is the main constituent of plaque? The answer came in the form of a 2001 publication in the *Annals of Biochemistry* (2001, 292: 234) and in an earlier publication in *Eiscosanoids* (1992, 5 : 17).

According to these studies, cholesterol esters that have become oxidised in the fatty acid chains (not in the steroid nucleus, as believed previously) are important components of plaque.

The main difference between these new findings and those of the earlier studies concerning "oxidised cholesterol", however, lies in the points in the cholesterol molecule where such oxidation takes place.

There are two sites in these cholesterol esters where oxidation can occur, namely in the steroid portion of the cholesterol molecule, or in the elongated side chains of the fatty acids found in the cholesterol esters.

Previously it was assumed that the oxidation occurs in the steroid portion of the molecule. This type of process cannot readily take place, however, and does not produce oxidation products that can lead to the restriction of arteries. Besides, such "oxidised cholesterol" cannot be shown analytically to be cholesterol *per se*. More recent studies have indicated that oxidation can also occur in the fatty acid chains of the cholesterol esters. Current thinking in this regard is mainly based on the findings of Prof. G. Spiteller and colleagues at the University of Bayreuth in Germany. These findings—which are of particular importance concerning many of the questions surrounding cancer and cardiac disease—can be summarised as follows:

- Polyunsaturated fatty acid (PUFA)—e.g. the w6 PUFA linoleic acid—is one of the most oxygen sensitive components of the cell. These PUFA occur in cells chiefly in the form of cholesterol esters and phospholipids in the cell membranes.
- During the storage and industrial processing (heating, filtration, etc.) of industrial oils such as sunflower oil—to "improve" their appearance—lipid peroxides are produced as a result of the nonenzymatic oxidation of cholesterol containing PUFA esters.
- These oxidised cholesterol esters (hereafter refered to as OCE) are incorporated into LDL (low density lipoproteins—the socalled "bad" cholesterol) and subsequently transported to the tissues, where they appear in the form of plaque.
- Thus we see that cholesterol *per se* is not the problem, and that the oxidation of cholesterol to form OCE, as so often occurs in the course of the preparation of our foods, is far more deserving of our attention (refer to the summarised versions by Dr. Spiteller in *Ann NY Acad Sc* 2005, 1043: 355).

This publication makes it clear that atherosclerosis is not a multifactorial process (more than one cause), but rather a multiplestep process in which lipoproteins are oxidised. The process whereby unchanged (i.e. nonoxidised) w6 fatty acid esters attain access to the cell membranes is a process that is strictly regulated. However, once the fatty acid esters become oxidised, this regulatory process ceases, with the result that the OCE are no longer removed systematically from the tissues and consequently accumulate as deposits.

Dr. Spiteller's conclusion is that there is only one cause of heart disease and that is the accumulation of defective w6 fatty acids (e.g. linoleic acid) in the artery walls.

All the negative results of clinical experiments based on the saturated fats—cholesterol theory as discussed in this book, can be interpreted on this basis.

Thus the clear connection between cardiac disease and cancer also becomes evident, following on the earlier studies of Prof. O. Warburg, as explained more fully in the book on cancer (*Cancer Diagnosed: What Now?*, Serfontein, W.J., Rosslyn Press, Pretoria, 2010). At once the fatty nature of plaque also becomes obvious.

CAN ATHEROSCLEROSIS AND THE FORMATION OF PLAQUE BE REVERSED?

Happily, the answer to this question is a clear "yes". This could occur under natural conditions, e.g. when a person changes his lifestyle and diet. It could also occur due to treatment. In this case there are two possibilities: firstly by way of intravenous chelation therapy (together with lifestyle and diet changes), or by means of oral nutritional methods, also referred to as nutritional arterial cleansing.

In practice, the effectiveness of these methods can be confirmed by means of objective testing, such as thermography (which measures infrared heat patterns) and pletismography, which registers blood flow patterns. In one study, these parameters were measured in the hands and feet of a group of men and women (average age 62 years) prior to and after treatment (6 weeks) by means of arterial cleansing. The results were as follows:

- Improved vascularity (blood perfusion), in hands 70% and in feet 86% (thermograph)
- Improved pulse volume, in hands 40% and in feet 50% (pletismograph)
- Improved plasticity of the arteries 47%. These figures indicate that arterial cleansing is a reality that can be objectively measured.

For anyone who has been afforded the opportunity to observe an open heart subsequent to a heart attack, the signs of inflammation in the affected heart are clearly visible.

WHAT ARE THE SYMPTOMS OF A HEART ATTACK?

The first symptom of a heart attack is usually sudden and acute chest pain. Patients describe it as a feeling of pressure or compression, like a heavy weight pressing down on the chest. This pain may then move to the arm, jawbone, neck or back. It may be accompanied by shortness of breath, lightheadedness, dizziness, feeling faint, sweatiness and nausea.

These symptoms may be different in men and women. In many women it may pass unnoticed, or they may experience a burning feeling in the abdominal area. Very often these symptoms are simply ignored, however, as they are not the typical chest pains of a heart attack. This can constitute an increased risk for the female patient.

WHAT SHOULD THE PATIENT DO IMMEDIATELY?

It is of cardinal importance that the patient should receive medical attention as soon as possible. For every minute that passes, a portion of the affected heart muscle is lost, reducing the chances of a complete recovery. Treatment will consist of medication to prevent the formation of clots and dissolve any clots that may already have formed. At the hospital the doctor will perform further tests to prove or disprove whether the patient did in fact have a heart attack, how serious it was and what treatment should be instituted.

FATS AND HEART DISEASE

It is important, with a view to the discussion to follow, for us to bear in mind that before the year 1900 (when heart disease was virtually unknown) a large portion of the diet consisted of unrefined carbohydrates and fats such as butter, lard and other animal fats. In Ireland, for example, a weekly consumption of 500 grams of butter was not uncommon (see more below).

There are, however, many people who maintain that there is in fact a connection between the consumption of fats and heart diseases. They claim that the low incidence of heart disease 80 years ago, compared with the high incidence at present, and the assumed connection that the consumption of fats has with heart disease, may be relayed to the fact that today we live in a world that is heavily polluted with environmental toxins, many of which are concentrated in our animal fats because of their solubility in fat.

This may be so, but this does not make animal fats *per se* a cause of heart disease.

REFINED FLOUR

Prior to the year 1900 most of the bread was baked with unrefined wheat flour which contained, inter alia, a variety of minerals and vitamins besides essential fatty acids and antioxidant tocopherols.

At about the turn of the previous century, roller mills were introduced in Europe, which simplified the milling process and particularly the separation of the various fractions of the flour. The immediate result was that flour could be milled finer and certain fractions could be easily removed. This could be achieved at far greater volumes and at a far faster rate than before. The refined wheat flour had a far higher glycemic index than the coarser flour. The result was *inter alia* that blood sugar levels rose faster and higher after the consumption of the refined flour, compared with the earlier consumption of coarser flour. This in turn gave rise to a significant increase in insulin resistance, accompanied by rising insulin levels in the consumer, which in turn gave rise to a higher risk of heart disease and diabetes.

Besides the greater refinement of the flour, it is today further treated with bleaching agents such as chlorine dioxide in order to "improve" the appearance. These bleaching agents then destroy any remaining traces of antioxidants and other nutritients that had previously been present in the wheat.

SOME IMPORTANT FACTS CONCERNING HEART DISEASE

- Diseases of the coronary heart vessels remain the major cause of death in the Western world, being responsible for over 40% of all deaths. Cancer is fast catching up, however. Together these two causes of death are responsible for 70 80% of all deaths in Western countries. This despite 50 years and billions of dollars spent on intensive medical research.

- In some countries, such as the USA and Australia, there has in fact been a decline in these figures during the past 20 years. The reasons for this are uncertain. Some researchers maintain that it has something to do with the fact that over this same period there was a 300% increase in the consumption of Vitamin C in the USA. In support of this, they point out those mammals such as guinea pigs, which manufacture their own Vitamin C endogenously (in the liver) do not suffer the same cardiovascular damage as humans who cannot manufacture their own Vitamin C. This will be discussed further below.

- Despite the fact that the role cholesterol plays in heart diseases is stressed by the medical fraternity, and particularly by the pharmaceutical industry, the truth is that almost 70% of all heart patients do not have elevated cholesterol levels (*Am J Med Sc* 1990, 299: 207). This crucial fact was conveniently disregarded in the past.

- At least 30 randomised clinical studies relating to the effect that the lowering of cholesterol levels by various methods (e.g. medication, diet) has had on the incidence of heart disease have been conducted, at a cost of over $1000 million. Not one of these studies has established unequivocally that the reduction of cholesterol saves lives. Despite this, a drug industry worth billions of rand has arisen and is marketing these drugs successfully to doctors and the public alike. Noone—least of all the popular press—mentions the volume of evidence indicating that it may be all be in vain

Plaque practically always develops at particular sites in the arterial system, and virtually never in the veinous system. It occurs mainly in arteries located near the heart, where pressure is highest and where, consequently, we may expect damage to the collagen and elastin structures of the arterial walls to be at its greatest. Vitamin C is crucial for the maintenance and repair of this tissue.

- About 50% of all patients who die of coronary heart disease do not have any of the recognised risk factors of the disease, including high cholesterol levels.

- Various population studies have shown that, although the lowering of blood cholesterol levels may hold certain benefits, such lowering of cholesterol levels is always accompanied by an increased risk of cancer. This matter will be discussed later in greater detail.
- Finally, it is important to recognise that about 80% of blood cholesterol is produced by the liver. Whenever the blood cholesterol levels are raised or lowered by an increase or decrease in the intake of cholesterol via the diet, the synthesis in the liver is adjusted accordingly, in order to keep blood levels more or less constant. The recommendation by so many doctors and dieticians to limit the intake of foods containing cholesterol, such as eggs, in order to prevent heart attacks, is simply incorrect.

This information is available in any good text book on biochemistry.

THEORIES ON HEART DISEASE: WHICH ONE IS RIGHT?

The fact that there are so many different theories concerning the possible causes of heart disease makes it very difficult to decide which one is correct, even for scientists who have busied themselves with this dilemma for years. For example, there is the Cholesterol Theory, claiming that heart disease is caused by high blood cholesterol levels. Then there is the Fat Theory, claiming that an excess of saturated fats and a shortage of polyunsaturated fats are the cause of elevated blood cholesterol levels; or the Homocysteine Theory which claims that elevated homocysteine levels as a result of the lack of certain vitamins is the cause of heart attacks; or the Oxidised Cholesterol theory, which states that cholesterol—particularly the cholesterol esters—become a risk once they have become oxidised; or the Free Radical and Heavy Metal Theory, which suggest that elevated levels of particular minerals—including iron—in the blood hold the answer; and last, but not the least, the Vascular Inflammation Theory.

Faced by this diversity of theories, deciding which one is true becomes a thorny issue. Despite this multiplicity, however, the medical profession has chosen to stick with one only, the Cholesterol Theory, and to apply it regardless. The fact that there is currently a mass of new evidence discounting this theory seems to have made no impression. We shall take a closer look at possible reasons for this later, but first let us consider a few of these theories.

THE FAT THEORY

According to this theory, too high a consumption of dietary fat leads to higher blood cholesterol levels, which in turn cause cholesterol to deposit on the walls of arteries. In time this becomes plaque and precipitates a heart attack. In addition, the assumption is that a high intake of dietary sugars may, in persons with a genetic tendency thereto, contribute to even higher cholesterol levels and consequently to a higher incidence of heart attacks.

A considerable amount of published information, however, contradicts the postulates of the Fat Theory. In the first place, there is more recent information concerning the composition of plaque. This has revealed that there are no saturated fats in plaque. The small amounts of cholesterol found in it cannot cause a heart attack, but are more likely to be a mechanism of the body aimed at repairing existing damage to the artery walls (*Lancet* 1994, 344: 1195).

At the onset of the previous century, when the incidence of heart attacks was very low, the customary diet contained large amounts of butter and lard (pork fat). According to current medical thinking, this should have caused a large number of heart attacks, but this was not the case. Margarine and commercialised sunflower seed oil, as we have come to know these in modern times, did not exist in those days.

Modern day margarines are prepared by a chemical process known as catalytic hydrogenation, using refined vegetable oils that have had their protective antioxidants (tocopherols) removed, and that contain many unnatural fats, such as transfatty acids. These margarines became popularised in about 1910 1920, at precisely the same time the rapid increase in heart diseases started to take place. Later it became evident that the transfatty acids in margarine are a contributing factor in the genesis of heart diseases and other health related problems. This gave rise to two issues: Firstly these products were no longer marketed under the name "margarine", but rather as "hydrogenated vegetable oils" (or something similar), which sounded better. Secondly, the manufacturers of margarine started producing a new type of margarine containing less transfatty acids, in an attempt to rescue their product. This "improved" product is still the result of processed vegetable and/or marine oils that have been hardened by alternative methods to make them seem more like butter. There is no proof that this product is less damaging in the long run than the previous forms of margarine.

Massive amounts of literature decrying the harmful effects of margarine have seen the light, but in spite of this, the Heart Foundation and many medical doctors and dieticians still recommend the use of margarine. The arguments they put forward in defense of these products still revolve around their seemingly unshakable faith that margarine and polyunsaturated fatty acids lower cholesterol levels and consequently also the risk of heart disease. More on this later.

THE ANTI-OXIDANT THEORY

During the 1970s Prof. Anderson of the University of Toronto in Canada presented evidence that poliunsaturated maize oil, of which the antioxidants had been removed, was harmful to the hearts of experimental animals. He then proceeded to relate these findings to the enormous increase in heart deaths as the use of polyunsaturated oils (including margarines) increased, and as the practice of eating refined grain in the form of bread became widespread.

In support of this evidence he cited the incidence of heart disease in Italy prior to and during and after the war, during the time span 1919 1948. In 1919 all refining and bleaching of wheat flour was forbidden in Italy, in order to reduce that country's dependence on imported wheat. This ban was maintained until 1946, and during this period there was no increase in the incidence of heart diseases in Italy. This was in contrast to many other countries, where an increase in the rate of heart deaths of up to 200% was experienced during the same period. Other findings supported the conclusions arrived at concerning the Italian experience. One study done in 1922 compared the incidence of heart disease in the south of France with that of Scotland. In many ways the two groups used in the study were the same; even their cholesterol levels were the same (6.0 mmol/L).

Despite this, the rate of heart deaths in Scotland was five times higher than that of France (Lancet, 20 June, 1992, p. 1423).

This difference was ascribed to the high level of the consumption of antioxidant rich wine in France—on average, 500 ml of red wine a day, which contained 100 mg of antioxidant bioflavonoids.

The antioxidant connection, and specifically the bioflavonoid antioxidants, was supported by the results of the Zutphen study in the Netherlands, in which a connection was established between bioflavonoid (quercetine) consumption and heart disease. This study found that men who consumed less than 10 mg of dietary quercetine per day had a risk of heart disease 200% higher than those whose intake was 30 mg per day or more. The chief sources of quercetine were apples, onions and tea. This higher consumption of quercetine was also found to be related to a reduction in deaths from other causes.

These and other similar studies strongly supported the relationship between heart health and the ingestion of antioxidants, but the exact mechanisms by which this takes place were uncertain. Besides, it was possible that the lower rate of heart deaths amongst those on the high quercetine diet could be the result of some other as yet unidentified factor, such as the intake of antiinflammatory substances. The only conclusion that is irrefutable, however, is that persons who eat more apples and onions have a lower risk of heart disease.

GOOD AND BAD FATS

Numerous studies have shown a connection between refined polyunsaturated oils (such as margarine and commercial sunflower oil) and heart disease. The reason behind this is that polyunsaturated fatty acids, by their very structure, are highly susceptible to oxidation by atmospheric oxygen. During this process they are converted into hydroperoxides, which in turn can give rise to the formation of dangerous free radicals, either as they are or by further degredation. These free radicals can damage cell membranes in critical tissues, such as the brain or the walls of arteries, thereby increasing the risk of heart disease. Pioneering work in this regard by Prof. O. Warburg (Nobel Prize winner) in 1929 1970 showed that damage to cell membranes caused intracellular oxygen pressure to decline to dangerously low levels within the cells, which is the real cause of cancer, and also of heart disease. (*J Cancer Res* 1925: 9,148).

Atherosclerosis (distinct from arteriosclerosis) occurs when lesions (plaque) occur on the inner walls of arteries, *inter alia* as a result of the damage caused by free radicals and/or hydroperoxides and by certain microorganisms. Antioxidants provided in sufficient quantities suppress this process.

Small amounts of certain essential fatty acids (w3 and w6 types) are needed for good health, and supplements such as fish oils, flax seed oil and unadulterated sunflower oil are often recommended to prevent shortages from occurring. The fatty acids present in these oils are also very susceptible to oxidation by atmospheric oxygen, which then gives rise to the same chain reaction that occurs when vegetable oils are refined, as discussed above. Such supplements should therefore be treated with great care to prevent oxidation.

This would include protection against atmospheric oxygen, and possibly the addition of an antioxidant such as Vitamin E.

THE "PRUDENT" DIET

The boundless faith displayed by the medical profession in cholesterol as the basic cause of heart diseases has led to attempts by the medical fraternity to design a diet that will reduce the levels of cholesterol in the blood. Noone has seen fit to question whether these statements (which are simply based on assumptions) are indeed true. Consequently, large sums of money and much time and effort have gone into designing a suitable diet, and then to confirming that it in fact does what is is intended to do.

The procedure used for evaluating this diet consisted in determining if it had any effect on the levels of cholesterol in the blood. At that time the possibility that some other factor was responsible for heart attacks was totally unthinkable.

This prompted the development of the socalled "Prudent" diet during the mid1950s. The term "Prudent" suggests and affirms the absolute faith that the medical profession had in the value of this diet to lower cholesterol levels, as well as to treat and to prevent heart disease.

What happened behind the scenes when this diet failed to meet expectations is quite amusing, if not, as some would put it, comical.

This diet focused sharply on the fat component. Medical policy required that the fat component of the Prudent diet should consist of at least two thirds polyunsaturated fats (margarine and vegetable oils). The other third consisted of saturated fats, such as butter.

The ultimate Prudent diet, in its final form, was proclaimed with great fanfare in the press, with the prospect that the solution to the heart problem was at hand. Most of the medical fraternity and the architects of medical opinion welcomed the diet with much enthusiasm and great expectation. Thousands of patients were immediately prescribed the new diet, and the public were likewise informed in order to prevent heart disease.

In our Faculty of Medicine, too, this diet was embraced with much acclaim.

There was, however, one prominent doctor who failed to share in the enthusiasm of the others. He was Dr. Paul White, personal cardiologist to the then President of the United States, Dwight Eisenhower. Dr White pointed out that he had been in practice as a cardiologist since 1921. During that period he saw a profound increase in the inci dence of heart disease, which had continued unabated through the time the Prudent diet had been followed by the public in general.

He saw his first case in 1931, at which time some of his colleagues had travelled long distances for the opportunity to observe this single case. He further pointed out that, prior to the 1930s, when heart attacks were virtually unknown, the general diet consisted largely of butter, fat and foods high in cholesterol.

Dr White's was a voice in the wilderness, however, and made no impression on the flood of prominent supporters of the Prudent diet, particularly after the voice of the mighty pharmaceutical industry ("Big Pharma") joined the chorus. The pharmaceutical industry at that stage was enthusiastically engaged in developing new cholesterol lowering drugs.

Further support for the Prudent diet came from the food industry, who were the main suppliers of the suddenly popularised polyunsaturated oils and margarines. These cheaper products soon started to replace butter in the market place, threatening to kill the butter industry.

The cumulative effect of the widespread publicity by the medical profession, supported by the powerful pharmaceutical and food industries, resulted in an increase in the consumption of polyunsaturated fats by the public of more that 300%. At the same time, butter virtually disappeared from the shelves of supermarkets.

This situation has prevailed more or less up to the present day, with the support of many doctors. Even the Heart Foundation is still recommending the use of margarine and polyunsaturated oils, maintaining that they are healthier.

It is significant to note that all the above took place, or is still taking place, without the Prudent diet ever having been subjected to a proper clinical trial.

However, as can be expected, the call to have the Prudent diet clinically assessed has progressively increased over time. This resulted in some of the clinical studies reported below.

Dr Wayne Martin is a prominent author on health matters in the USA. The following is a brief account of his report on what went on behind the scenes.

THE JOLIFFE ANTICORONARY CLINICAL STUDY

This study was organized by Dr. Joliffe in New York, partly as a result of the fact that he was himself seriously ill, suffering from diabetes and heart disease. Joliffe was confined to a wheelchair, with vascular lesions of the eyes and ulcers in one foot, due to complications arising from his diabetes. He was convinced that the experiment he had planned for the Prudent diet would bring the solution to his own health problems. Consequently, he arranged for himself to join the trial as a member of the active trial group which was to be compared with the control group which was on a normal diet. He invited teachers and lecturers from various colleges in New York to join him in the treatment group.

The control group consisted of prosperous businessmen from New York society, who lived on the typical high fat, high cholesterol diet of the affluent. This diet provided a high level of saturated fats, in contrast to the Prudent diet. In this manner it was hoped to demonstrate once and for all the harmful effects of a diet high in saturated fats.

The selection of the test group and the control group from two different sections of society could be seen as a weakness in the study design. In this manner, the test could be seen to have been designed with the specific intent of displaying—and emphasising—the benefits of the Prudent diet over the traditional American diet.

The study ran over a period of 6 years, at the end of which the results were published in JAMA in 1966. As expected, it was found that the cholesterol levels of the test group had declined by 10%, when compared with the control group.

Based on this fact alone, the study was declared a resounding success by many doctors and by the popular press, and the Prudent diet was reaffirmed as the manner in which the epidemic of heart diseases could be successfully combated.

Noone considered whether the lowering of cholesterol levels was indeed synonymous with the increase of lifespan.

The conviction that high cholesterol levels were the absolute cause of heart disease was so deeply ingrained that it was unthinkable that this could perhaps not be true. This perception persists in the minds of many medical doctors, and in much of the public at large, even today, thanks to the continued propaganda by the popular press, and especially the pharmaceutical industry.

The results did reveal the shocking fact, however, that the number of heart deaths in Dr Joliffe's two groups was precisely the opposite of what they had expected. Eight patients in the Prudent diet group died during the study, while there were no deaths in the control group.

This fact was not made known, however.

This, as well as the fact that Dr Joliffe himself died shortly afterwards, was not revealed. The number of unexpected deaths in the test group was ascribed to chance, while Dr Joliffe's death was put down to his advanced diabetic condition.

The reaction within the inner circles of the medical profession was that the experiment hab been a success after all, considering the significant lowering of cholesterol levels that were seen. A decision was taken to follow it up immediately with a further trial, using a far larger number of participants, consisting of one million patients. This never materialised.

FURTHER PROSPECTIVE CLINICAL STUDIES

NATIONAL DIET HEART STUDY

The new experiment was to be known as the "National Diet Heart Study", under the leadership of the National Heart Institute, funded by the American government. Dr. Irvine Page of the Cleveland Clinic was appointed leader of the new study group.

Dr. Martin recalls in an entertaining manner the discussion he had with Dr. Page (*Arch Int Med* 1992, 152:1371). Dr. Page was himself the victim of a heart attack, and he was convinced that the Prudent diet would prevent a recurrence.

The new experiment was planned on a grand scale. Food depots were established in 5 large cities where participants in the study could get their free supply of food with the correct composition, e.g. doughnuts prepared in polyunsaturated fatty acids, and meat from which all fat had been removed. The control group followed the normal American diet.

Before starting with the main experiment of one million patients, it was wisely decided to do a trial run with only 2 000 men (ages 45 54 years). These were divided into 2 random groups, in order to eliminate the possibility that the results could be caused by other extraneous factors. This pretest was also run over a period of 6 years and the results were published in *Circulation* magazine.

As expected, there was a reduction of blood cholesterol levels of 6.5 to 5.8 mmol/L (10.7%) in the test group, which prompted one group of cardiologists to declare the study a success, and to insist on the immediate institution of the main trial.

However, no clinical advantage over the control group could be demonastrated in the smaller preliminary trial group.

Another group of cardiologists—probably because of this—were hesitant to begin such a large undertaking on the basis of the available information. Both the number of heart deaths and the number of nonheart related deaths were identical in both the groups. In the end the larger study was cancelled—"due to the high cost factor".

The public, as well as the professional community, were not informed that the test group showed no clinical advantage over the control group.

Nonetheless, and on similar other evidence, we still hear medical doctors, dieticians and even the Heart Foundation promoting the merits of margarine and polyunsaturated fats for the prevention of heart attacks. Not only is there no underlying clinical support for such a viewpoint, there is evidence that such a diet may increase the risk of heart disease.

POPULATION STUDIES

The failure of the two studies described above to produce clinical evidence of any advantage to be gained from the Prudent diet has been regarded by some cardiologists as the result of failings in the design of the particular trials. The boundless enthusiasm of some cardiologists for the the Prudent diet (needless to say, with the keen support of the pharmaceutical industry) led to new avenues being investigated in search of support for the Prudent diet. One novel approach was to compare the level of heart attacks in various population groups with differing dietary patterns. In this manner support could possibly obtained for the polyunsaturated fat theory.

THE BOSTON—IRELAND BROTHERS STUDY

At that time the diet of persons living in the Boston area of the USA was generally quite close to the Prudent diet, probably due to the active promotion by doctors. On the other hand, Ireland was predominantly a dairynation, *inter alia* because of legislation protecting butter against the cheaper imported polyunsaturated oils and margarines. As a result, the average butter consumption of the Irish was some 500g of butter per week per person, while their consumption of polyunsaturated oils and margarine was almost zero. This situation afforded an ideal opportunity to compare the incidence of coronary heart disease in the two populations, and to cast further light on the advantages or otherwise of polyunsaturated oils (World Rev Nut Diet 1970, 12: 142).

Dr Stare, who organised the study, managed to identify families in Ireland of which one brother still resided in Ireland while another brother had emigrated to Boston in America. The belief existed that the incidence of heart disease among the brothers in Ireland would be far higher than among the Boston brothers.

> *Precisely the opposite then became evident. The Boston brothers had a far higher rate of heart diseases than their Irish brothers (Lancet, Aug. 1973, p 298).*

This was front page news in the USA, and somewhat uncomfortable for the cardiologists. They rationalised the finding as being the result of the far more active lifestyle of the Irish, who had to walk wherever they wanted to go. This could indeed be partly true, but the test results still pointed to the fact that high fat intakes in the form of butter do not necessarily cause heart attacks.

THE ROSETO STUDY

Roseto was a small town in Pennsylvania, USA, with almost 100% Italian inhabitants. It was a known fact that the incidence of heart attacks was lower in Italy, and also in Roseto, than elsewhere. It was also a known fact that the incidence of heart attacks in Roseto was lower than that in the neighbouring districts in Pennsylvania, which had a high percentage of Dutch residents. The eating habits in these two populations were very dissimilar. The Italians were mostly welloff, and their diet consisted largely of high fat meat balls and a lot of Italian cheeses, containing hardly any polyunsaturated fats. The diet of their Dutch neighbours, on the other hand, followed the typical American dietary pattern, which was similar to the Prudent diet. This situation presented an ideal opportunity to study the effect of the two different diets on heart disease.

Prof Wolf of the University of Oklahoma launched just such a study (*Trans Am Climatol Assoc* 1973, 85: 100). The results indicated that the incidence of heart disease among the residents of Roseto, with the high percentage of saturated fats in their diet, was about one third lower than the average for the rest of America.

Once again the cardiologists did not anticipate such an outcome and declared that the differences observed were due to the fact that the Italians were mostly members of a single large family, which would reduce their stress levels.

Nonetheless, it can be stated that the consumption of a diet high in fats does not necessarily lead to an increased risk of heart attacks. This also correlates with the findings of other studies.

THE INDIAN POPULATION STUDY

Dr Malhotra of India undertook a study of heart diseases in two Indian population groups with almost directly opposite dietary habits (*Am J Clin Nutr.* May 1967, p 452). One group lived in the north of India where there was an abnormally high consumption of butter in the form of ghee (clarified butter). The incidence of heart diseases among this group—which was relatively affluent—was known to be very low.

The second group consisted of relatively poor people in the south of India, whose diet—probably due to economic reasons—corresponded to a large extent with the Prudent diet. The mainly fat component in their diet consisted of polyunsaturated oils in the form of peanut oil and the margarine made of this oil. They consumed almost no saturated fats.

> *The results of this study showed that there were some 15% more heart attacks in the Prudent diet group than in the group with the high butter consumption.*

Once again, this was diametrically opposite to what the cardiologists would have predicted. Later reports revealed, however, that there was a significant increase in the number of heart deaths in the north—probably due to economic reasons—when butter was replaced with the cheaper polyunsaturated oils and margarine (*Lancet* Nov. 1987, p 1144).

FURTHER CHOLESTEROL-HEART DISEASE

CLINICAL STUDIES

THE "MULTIPLE RISK FACTOR INTERVENTION STUDY" (MRFIT)

This was a multiple intervention study covering the effect on the incidence of heart disease of a variety of heart risk factors. The study cost $175 million and involved 28 medical centres and 250 researchers.

A test group of men with a high heart risk rate was selected from a population of 361 662 men. In this manner 12 866 men in the age group 35 37 years old were randomly assigned to either the test group or the control group. The risk factors that were to be modified in the test group were hypertension and smoking. They were also given advice on diet, aimed at reducing cholesterol.

After arranging the implication of these interventions in the two groups, the patients were monitored for 7 years. The following results were recorded: cholesterol intake from food was reduced by 42% and a reduction of 28% in saturated fats intake were recorded in the experimental group.

A moderate lowering of blood cholesterol levels in the patients in the experimental group was achieved, but there was no difference in total deaths, particularly heart related deaths, between the two groups.

The authors of this study referred to these results as "disappointing". The final conclusion was that "the total results indicate no beneficial effect on the incidence of coronary heart disease or mortality in this multiple intervention study" in the intervention group compared to the control group.

THE PHYSICIANS' HEALTH STUDY

In the USA, 51 259 male physicians participated in this study. The participants periodically submitted responses to questionnaires regarding their diet, lifestyle and any changes to their state of health.

> *An important finding of this study was that the daily intake of aspirin reduced heart attacks by 55%.*

There were complete reports by 43 732 participants concerning the results that were obtained on the other parameters of the study. These showed that total fat intake and the intake of specific types of fat and cholesterol had no effect on the incidence of strokes and heart attacks. The conclusion was therefore that a diet based on the standard food pyramid (which was based on the Prudent diet) did not reduce the incidence of heart disease, stroke or cancer.

THE FRAMINGHAM STUDY

This was the largest and most influential heart study of all time. It was performed on all the inhabitants (5 000) of a small town (Framingham) in Massachusetts, USA. It was started in 1975 and has now been running for 35 years.

This was not a controlled study, with a test group and a control group, as in the case of the studies cited above. This was purely an observational study, which documented living habits in terms of parameters that are regarded as important for heart patients. These included lifestyle, diet, blood pressure and blood cholesterol. There were large individual differences in the daily intake of cholesterol, which, however, had little effect on the fluctuation of blood cholesterol levels.

> *This serves to underline the wellknown biochemical fact that there is no connection between diet cholesterol and blood cholesterol levels.*

In the light of this, it is difficult to understand that there are still medical doctors and dieticians who assert that eggs are undesirable in the diet of heart patients due to the high cholesterol levels in eggs.

The next matter of importance was the connection between saturated fats in the diet and blood cholesterol levels. Once again it came to the fore that there is no connection between the intake of saturated fats and blood cholesterol levels. Despite the findings of this prestigious study (and of others with the same conclusions), the medical fraternity—and the Heart Foundation—still persist in cautioning against the intake of fats in the diet as being a possible cause of heart disease.

Another remarkable and perhaps valuable finding of the study was that the daily intake of a low dose of aspirin resulted in a significant reduction in the incidence of coronary heart disease

In December 1997, in a followup report on the Framingham study, the amazing result was revealed that an increase in the intake of saturated fats even resulted in a lowering of the incidence of strokes.

This conclusion, which is in direct conflict with the philosophy of the majority of medical researchers and medical doctors, came as a severe shock. What was remarkable in this study, as in other similar studies that contradict the expectations of medical researchers, is that these researchers then resorted to farfetched "justifications" as to why the findings are in conflict with their expectations. In this case they speculated that the fatty diet led to the early death due to heart attacks of the older participants in the study of heart attacks before they could suffer a stroke!

Outrageous statements such as these demonstrate the determination of the investigators that the study results should support the low fat, low cholesterol diet theory.

Subsequently the investigators were obliged to concede that this study didn't succeed in providing support for the cholesterol theory or for the prudent diet.

The end conclusion of the Framingham study—after 35 years of expensive research and investment—was therefore that there is no connection between the intake of fats and coronary heart disease.

This conclusion is supported by the results of other similar studies, such as the MRTIT study, the Physicians' Health study, and the Womens' Health study, all of which were briefly discussed above.

Collectively these studies have shown that

- Reduced intake of cholesterol in the diet has no effect on the incidence of heart disease
- A lowfat diet doesn't lower the risk of heart disease, and

- A daily dose of aspirin does lower the risk of heart disease

It is astounding that the message contained in these studies has not penetrated medical thinking. The medical authorities that designed and ran the study were so convinced that there must be a connection between cholesterol and heart disease that they were not prepared to accept any finding that was in conflict with this view. They preferred to justify the divergent results in some other way, rather than accept the inevitable conclusion that cholesterol is not involved, and that the solution should rather be sought in the direction suggested by the aspirin effect, namely that inflammation should be further investigated as the basic cause of heart disease.

The public, the medical world, and the pharmaceutical and food industries were so firmly convinced that cholesterol was indeed the big bad wolf, that the scientific facts mentioned above could not turn this saga around, especially after these industries had invested vast sums of money in support of this view, and in establishing it in the minds of the public.

THE WOMEN'S HEALTH INITATIVE STUDY

This study was performed on 48 835 postmenopausal women at a cost of $415 million. The participants were randomly divided into two equal groups, of which the one was to serve as control (no intervention). The active group received advice regarding behaviour modification, as well as directives regarding their diet, aimed at reducing their fat consumption by 20% calories. Participants were also advised to include fruit and vegetables (5 portions of each daily), and grains (6 portions per day) in their food. This diet was approximately the same as the socalled food pyramid, which had been widely promoted by the American government and elsewhere in the world.

After an average followup period of 8.1 years, there was no reduction in heart disease, strokes or cancer in the test group, as compared with the control group.

The collective results of a number of studies (some of which have been briefly discussed above) indicate that the polyunsaturated oils and margarine are not only ineffective for preventing heart disease, but may actually cause them.

Granted, these oils and margarines do lower blood cholesterol levels, but despite this they do not lower the risk of heart attacks, nor do they reduce the number of deaths. This casts doubt once again on the connection between cholesterol and heart risk, as it had been accepted by almost everyone, and is still a belief of many. Besides this, we must bear in mind that 70% of heart patients do not have elevated levels of cholesterol or of blood fats previouslly discussed.

It is therefore fundamentally wrong to lower the cholesterol levels of everyone who is at risk of having a heart attack, especially not by the use of cholesterol lowering medication.

Meanwhile, we should ask how it is possible that the fat theory of heart disease could endure so long in the face of evidence that has been available since 1960 that it is in error in its present form.

This reminds one of what Huxley once said:

> *the great tragedy of science is the slaying of a beautiful hypothesis by an ugly fact.*

I propose that there are at least two reasons for the professional unwillingness to accept the above results. Firstly, it reflects the power of the money wielded by the pharmaceutical and food industries to influence the thinking of the medical world and the public. One has to bear in mind that the turnover of a single cholesterol lowering drug in the USA alone is as much as $13 billion per annum. This gives us an idea of the extent of financial involvement here, and why these money moguls would be prepared to sacrifice the lives of people and disregard the evidence.

Secondly, I propose that certain opinion leaders, who years ago took a decisive stand in favour of the cholesterol theory, are finding it extremely difficult to do a complete turnaround in public without losing face. Medical thinking is largely determined by opinion leaders, who are mostly older, revered members of the medical and scientific communities. Many of these opinion leaders also have connections with the pharmaceutical industry.

WHAT PRECISELY IS THE CHOLESTEROL THEORY?

The wellknown scientific author, H L Mencken, once said:

> *For every complex problem there is usually a solution that is simple and easy to comprehend and wrong.*

There are very few scientific arenas where this truth is more applicable than in the cholesterolheart disease problem. Let us hasten to add that, precisely because the cholesterolheart disease connection seemed so easy to understand, it attracted large numbers of supporters, among professionals and novices alike. It also caught the attention of the large pharmaceutical companies, because this theory lent itself *par excellence* to the development of new drugs, of which the proposed function would also be "simple and easy to comprehend". Need we point out that, in most cases, new truths were to emerge around these "easy and understandable" solutions that were not so simple, albeit they were closer to the truth?

What is readily understandable, however, is the fact that, once the large pharmaceutical companies became involved, it was extremely difficult for them to change direction, due to the enormous sums of money involved in the development of the new products.

> *This is the exact scenario that took place in the case of the cholesterolheart disease question.*

The cholesterol theory postulates that saturated animal fats in the diet cause elevated blood cholesterol levels by which the precipitation of cholesterol in the walls of the arteries is increased. This in turn leads to the accumulation of plaque, which consists of deposits in the artery walls of heart patients. Few other theories—including the polyunsaturated margarine saga—have provoked more debate and controversy in medical circles.

Today many researchers believe that saturated fats can only increase the blood cholesterol levels if there is also a high intake of refined carbohydrates. The question remains, however, whether it is indeed the cholesterol *per se* which is responsible for the heart attacks under these conditions.

In the past, researchers have erred in clinical trials by changing only one variable (such as the cholesterol in the example above) and then holding it solely responsible for the observed clinical results. In turn, this error can often be referred back to the researcher's lack of insight into statistics.

At the present time the medical profession still solidly supports the saturated fatscholesterol theory as originally formulated in the 1960s. The result is that a cholesterol lowering drug is usually prescribed for every patient with a heart problem. This senseless and dangerous practice will be discussed below.

The statins are the latest class of cholesterol lowering medicines that are very effective in lowering blood cholesterol levels, and consequently these are very popular amongst medical doctors, as most of them still believe that cholesterol is the cause of heart attacks. Granted, there are individual studies that indicate that these drugs hold certain short term benefits in terms of patient survival. This does not automatically mean that the observed clinical effects (e.g. fewer heart attacks) are necessarily the result of lower cholesterol levels. And what are often ignored is the serious side effects that these drugs have (see below).

There can be little doubt that, in population studies, there is a connection between blood cholesterol levels and the incidence of heart diseases. This connection need not necessarily be causative, however. The high cholesterol levels may actually indicate metabolic disturbances, which may be the true cause of the disease. In conditions such as these it would be wrong in principle to choose a cholesterol lowering medication (e.g. a statin) as the primary therapeutic approach.

WHAT SHOULD WE DEDUCE FROM THIS?

The combined results of a large number of studies (some of which have been briefly dealt with above) have indicated that the polyunsaturated diet is not only ineffective in preventing heart attacks, but it may actually cause heart attacks.

Granted, these oils and margarines do lower blood cholesterol levels, but notwithstanding this, they do not reduce the risk of heart attacks, and they do not reduce the number of deaths. This questions once more the connection between cholesterol and heart risk, which has been so widely accepted by cardiologists and doctors in the past. Besides this, we must recall that some 70% of heart attack patients do not have elevated levels of cholesterol or any other blood fats. It would therefore be fundamentally wrong to lower the cholesterol level of any patient who is at risk of having a heart attack, and especially not by administering cholesterol lowering medication. More about this later.

Meanwhile, we still ask the question: how is it possible that the fat theory of heart disease could endure so long in spite of the fact that since 1960 evidence has been available that this theory—in its present form—is wrong?

I propose that at least two reasons for this are at hand. Firstly, it reflects the influence that the financially powerful pharmaceutical and food industries have on medical thinking and on the public at large. Bear in mind that the turnover of a single cholesterol lowering drug in the USA alone is in excess of $13 billion per annum. This figure gives us some idea of what is actually involved here, and why these financial moguls are prepared to sacrifice the lives of people as they chase after these lage financial gains.

Secondly, I put it to you that some prominent opinion formers who took a strong stand in favour of the cholesterol theory many years ago now find it extremely difficult to switch to the opposite view without losing face. Medical thinking is mostly shaped by opinion leaders, consisting mostly of highly honoured, older members of the medical and scientific community. Many of these opinion leaders also have ties with the pharmaceutical industry.

THE INSTABILITY OF FATTY ACID ESTERS AND THE CONNECTION BETWEEN CANCER AND HEART DISEASES

Recent work done by Prof. B. Peskin and associates in the USA focused attention once again on the research done by Prof. O. Warburg of Germany on cancer during the period 1920 1970 (*Cancer Res* 1979, 39:1726). Warburg found that if the intracellular oxygen level declines by more than 35%, normal cells start fermenting (utilising glucose without oxygen to produce energy) instead of the normal production of energy by means of respiration (production of energy from glucose using oxygen). During this process the cells become cancerous. It also became evident that certain fatty acids (unadulterated linoleic acid that occurs in natural sunflower oil) as constituent of the cell membranes, control the process of the normal entry of oxygen into the cells. These fatty acids are usually present as esters (condensation products) of cholesterol, but during the commercial processing of sunflower oil, oxidation of the fatty acid chains in the esters occurs, with the result that the fatty acid molecules lose their ability to transfer oxygen from the blood to the inside of the cells.

This has extremely important implications regarding the cancer problem, but it also has a role to play in heart diseases, as indicated in the research done by Prof Spiteller.

> *Prof Spiteller found that these unnatural adulterated) fatty acid esters are important constituents of plaque (Annals NY Acad Sc 2005, 1043: 355).*

Spiteller makes it plain that in his view there is only one cause of coronary heart disease, and that is the accumulation in the cells of the artery walls of these adulterated derivatives of linoleic acid.

> *He further emphasises that the principal component of arterial plaque is made up of the partially adulterated esters of linoleic acid, and that this is also present in cancer cells.*

> *This also reveals the long sought after connection between cancer and heart disease.*

It is a well known fact that when cholesterol levels are reduced, the risk of cancer increases. In terms of the findings of Prof. Spiteller, we can now understand why this is so. These findings by Prof. Spiteller have been confimed by other researchers (*Ann Bioch* 2001, 292: 234).

In contrast to the popular view, it is not cholesterol *per se* that deposits in the artery wall during the process of atherosclerosis, but in fact the products of the oxidised side chains of the cholesterol esters.

Then it immediately becomes clear why simply reducing the levels of blood cholesterol is not an effective way to prevent heart disease. We should rather be preventing the oxidation of the cholesterol esters, which in practice means that we should be avoiding the oxidation of sunflower oil and other similar products, which happens when they are "purified" industrially, involving the processes of filtration, oxidation, discolouring, etc. to make them look better.

CHOLESTEROL LOWERING DRUGS

During the past few decades, various cholesterol reducing drugs have been developed in an attempt to reduce the rapidly growing number of heart deaths, in spite of the fact that no irrefutable proof exists that the lowering of cholesterol levels is effective in achieving this. Nonetheless, these drugs are still being prescribed by doctors and cardiologists at an alarming rate.

The Lipid Research Clinics Coronary Prevention Trial (costing $175 m) is one example of the clinical effects associated with druginduced cholesterol reduction. The trial did show a mild reduction in the number of heart deaths in the short term, but simultaneously the total mortality figures increased from other causes, such as cancer (*BMJ* 1984, 288:424). There was no difference in total mortality between the trial and control groups due to the increased cancer incidence. The increase in cancer deaths is understandable, in the light of what has been said above regarding the oxidation of the fatty acid chains in the cholesterol esters.

Since the 1980s a new group of very effective cholesterol reducing agents, known as statins, have come onto the market. The question whether they carry any true benefits for the patient, remains yet unanswered. Currently the statins are among the most frequently prescribed medications.

Some studies have indicated that they do reduce the number of heart deaths in the short term. The Scandinavian Simastatin Survival Study (S4 study) (*Lancet* 1994, 344: 1383) is one of the most significant of these studies. The results showed that Simvastatin (a popular statin) not only reduces cholesterol effectively in patients with high cholesterol levels, but that the treatment is also clinically of benefit in the short term (5 years). The rate of survival after 5 years was 30% higher for the treatment group than for the control group. Other similar studies gave much the same results, including one done on healthy persons with high cholesterol levels.

Collectively, these results confirmed in the minds of many doctors that the lowering of cholesterol levels was indeed the most effective means of reducing heart attacks. The result was that the use of statins in treating heart patients became more or less standard practice. Few doctors took note of the fact that over 30 other studies indicated the direct opposite. This led to the idea that the proven benefits of the statins had nothing to do with their cholesterol lowering effect. This view was reinforced by a further study (*Lancet* 1996, p 781), and there was talk of the "extra lipid effects" of the statins. This referred to the observed stabilising effect of statins on plaque deposits, in which the tendency of such deposits to rupture and cause a heart attack was said to be reduced. There was also a possibility that statins may have antioxidant properties. All the above led to the popularity of the statins rising to unprecedented heights. In the ensuing atmosphere of euphoria, the possible negative aspects of the statins were overlooked. Some of these included serious side effects, and the slumbering question remained unanswered, whether they bring any real benefits for the patient. Further, the possibility had been overlooked, that any benefits the statins provided were probably not linked to their cholesterol reducing effects, and further, that the use of patient cholesterol levels as an indicator and guide for the use of statins could be erroneous.

THE STATINS: AN EPILOGUE

As early as 1984, during a congress of the Cholesterol Consensus Conference, guidelines concerning "safe cholesterol levels" were established. It was determined that both men and women should have blood cholesterol levels below 5.16 mmol/L, and that anyone presenting with levels above this limit should immediately be treated with a statin. It is significant to note that for each 0.1 mmol/L that this critical level is lowered, a few hundred thousand new patients are added to the numbers of those requiring statins, which translates into an additional income of millions of dollars for the pharmaceutical industry. It came as no surprise, therefore, when this critical level was subsequently lowered to 4.6 mmol/L, and some time later, to 4.4 mmol/L. This meant millions of extra dollars in profit for the pharmaceutical giants. What was not acknowledged, however, is that these reduced cholesterol levels significantly increased the patient's chances of developing cancer or a stroke. They also neglected to point out the importance of cholesterol in the body's maintenance system. Cholesterol is essential for the maintenance of all cell membranes, for the synthesis of the sex hormones and other steroids, besides many other biological functions.

There are many ways in which medical doctors (most of whom have little or no knowledge of statistics) can be misled by an industry that has a vested interest in the medications market. The following example, cited by Dr. Lundell, a former cardiac physician, in his book, supports this view point.

In a television programme about the statin Lipitor, a certain Dr. Jarvik stated that Lipitor reduced the incidence of heart attacks by 36%. To support this statement, Dr. Jarvis quoted the results of a study done on Lipitor with thousands of patients, which indicated that heart attacks in the control group over the specific period was 3%, while only 2% of the Lipitor group suffered heart attacks. On the grounds of this, Dr Jarvis deduced that Lipitor reduced the incidence of heart attacks by 36%! This is a colossal statistical blunder. Statistics require that in studies of this nature, the numbers of patients must be taken into condideration in the calculations.

According to the above figures, 100 patients must be treated with Lipitor for 3.5 years in order to prevent one heart attack (3% 2%). This implies that 99 out of the 100 Lipitor users received no benefit from the use of this medication.

There is a constant in statistics known as the "NNT", or "number necessary to treat". The NNT indicates the number of persons that have to be treated in order to prevent one adverse event. The NNT for most of the antibiotics is about 1.1, which means that of every 11 patients who receive treatment, 10 will benefit from it. The above figures indicate that in the case of Lipitor, 100 patients must be treated for 3.5 years to prevent one heart attack!

> *Various other scientific publications have indicated that the NNT for statins is not 100, but rather 250.*

This means that 249 out of every 250 patients who have been treated with statins will derive no benefit from the treatment.

Prof J R Hoffman, professor in clinical medicine at the University of California, had the following to say about this:

> *If there are 250 persons in a room, who are given the choice of paying more than $1000 per annum for a medicine that they have to use daily, that will give them diarrhoea and muscular pains, knowing that 249 of them will derive no benefit from this, how many of them would accept the offer?*

Clearly very few!

Another scholar in this field noted that this type of benefit was comparable to a lottery—you have practically no chance of winning.

THE ROLE OF THE PHARMACEUTICAL COMPANIES

The pharmaceutical companies have a moral responsibility towards their shareholders to show a reasonable profit. Besides this, we need them to develop new medications, as they are financially capable of doing this. Their original calling was to develop effective medicines at a reasonable price.

However, when some of them become involved in profiteering, and stoop to promoting products by subtle means or by exaggerating their benefits, and when they start infiltrating medical institutions in a doubtful manner, the stage is set for large scale corruption and malpractice.

I wish to make it quite clear that, in my view, the medical doctors who prescribe statins are not corrupt. They are, however, obliged to function within a particular system, which has been set up by the opinion leaders and sometimes by the heads of some of the pharmaceutical companies. The majority of medical doctors are honest and hardworking, who strive to do the best they can for their patients, within the system they have to work in.

PRESSURE ON THE MEDICAL PROFESSION

There are many responsible doctors who are at least partly aware of what is being dealt with in this book. They hesitate to express their opinions in public, however, because many of the official bodies and organisations that exercise control over the marketing of medicines, and over official medical policies do not take kindly to being criticised in public. They often use coercion to express their displeasure at being criticised, by uttering thinly veiled threats of legal action, and by spreading false statements. A telling example of this has been cited by Dr. H. Barry of the Michigan State University College of Medicine. He commented on the National Cholesterol Education Program (NCEP) and the manner in which it gives guidance regarding cholesterol and heart diseases. Readers will recall that the NCEP is the body in America that must give guidance regarding the problem of heart diseases. This is also the body that determined the maximum acceptable levels of blood cholesterol, as referred to above.

As their name implies, their main object is to indicate how cholesterol is to be brought under control. Noone in this group ever questioned whether cholesterol is indeed involved as a cause of heart diseases, because this is accepted as selfevident in the medical world.

Dr Barry and 34 other professionals lodged an official objection with the National Institute of Health (NIH) stating that the facts on which the NCEP based their guidelines were very vague, and that the NCEP panel were biased because 8 of the 9 members had interests in the pharmaceutical industry.

In support of this objection, they cited the opinion of Prof. R. Hayward (Professor in Internal Medicine at the Medical School of the University of Michigan). He had stated that the current evidence calls for the entire concept of the involvement of LDL (i.e. cholesterol) as a cause of heart disease to be abandoned. In other words, cholesterol is of no importance.

In response, the NCEP threatened legal action in a most uncivil manner, more befitting extremists, and certainly not to be expected of an official body such as the NCEP, nor from objective and unbiased scientists.

Other researchers pointed out, and quite rightly so, that if only a fraction of the thousands of millions of dollars that had been expended on studies regarding cholesterol as well as on medications and on doctors' consultations could have been applied to informing the public concerning diet, exercising and the reduction of body mass, everyone would have been far healthier.

Dr. Lundell is the former Head of Staff and Surgery at the Banner Heart Hospital in Mesa, Arizona, USA. He had practised cardiac surgery for 25 years, performing over 5 000 open heart operations during that period.

In a move that caused him great anguish, he felt obliged one day to simply close his practice, because he could no longer see his way clear to participate in the cholesterol mania and everything it brought with it in terms of the role of surgery as a means of dealing with heart disease. He then proceeded, following the dictates of his convictions concerning the truth about the heart challenge, to document this in his book entitled *The Great Cholesterol Lie* (ISBN 9780979034015).

> *His approach to heart disease was based entirely on his experience in the operating theatre.*

In that book, which contains very fundamental truths concerning heart disease and cholesterol, he lays great emphasis on the role of arterial inflammation in atherosclerosis. I strongly recommend the reader to study Dr. Lundell's book in detail, and to evaluate the whole question of the true causes of heart disease in terms of what is contained in his book, as well as on what is to be discussed below. More detail, as well as important preventative procedures that can be performed, will be discussed later.

From the above brief discussion it becomes clear that the debate on heart disease and cholesterol is no longer based on scientific facts, and that some participants in this debate do so with a variety of ulterior motives.

THE HARMFUL EFFECTS
OF STATINS

It came as a great shock to millions of doctors and patients when the wellknown pharmaceutical company Bayer announced in 2002 that they would be withdrawing the cholesterol lowering statin Cervastatin ("Baycol") from the market with immediate effect.

The reason put forward for this decision was the growing number of reports concerning the side effects of this medication, including, muscular pains and weakness (rhabdomyolysis), particularly if the medicine is taken together with other cholesterol lowering drugs.

Rhabdomyolysis is otherwise a very rare but potentially life threatening condition that manifests initially as muscular pain, but can develop into kidney failure and even death. Approximately 53 such cases were reported against Baycol before it was withdrawn.

Baycol was one of 5 different statins on the South African market at that time. Apparently the other statins are less toxic than Baycol.

Nevertheless, the European Medicines Evaluation Agency (EMEA) decided to reevaluate all statins in 2001.

Meanwhile, statins are being prescribed on a large scale—almost always for their cholesterol lowering effect (for which they are very effective) and not on the basis of patient mortality, although there are some clinical studies that indicate possible short term benefits. Not a single long term study has as yet been undertaken with statins.

The effect of statins on Q10 blood levels (especially in the mitochondria) is however a source of much concern.

The mitochondria are structures within the cell where energy is produced from carbohydrates and fats. For this process coenzyme Q10 is needed. The biochemical process in which Q10 is produced in the body starts with acetic acid and proceeds via mevalonic acid, after which the process divides into 2 branches. The one branch leads to Q10, and the other to cholesterol. The statins suppress an enzyme higher up in the chain, and by inhibiting this enzyme they suppress the synthesis of both Q10 and cholesterol. While the lowering of cholesterol is the desired effect of the statins, the simultaneous suppression of the synthesis of Q10 is highly undesirable, but unavoidable. Many of the long term side effects of statins can be referred back to the low Q10 levels they cause. There are many publications confirming the effect of lowered Q10 levels by the use of statins. Such a shortage of Q10 in the heart muscle gives rise to a reduction of energy production in the heart muscle. The heart then becomes progressively disabled and less blood can be pumped, to the point where a heart transplant may be the only way to save a patient's life. This condition is known as cardiomyopathy.

THE STATINS: A SUMMARY

There are benefits to be derived from using statins for heart patients, but these benefits apparently have nothing to do with their cholesterol lowering qualities. These benefits are observable in heart patients long before the reduction of cholesterol takes place; therefor the benefits are independent of the reduction of cholesterol.

The following facts concerning the statins are, however, accepted:

- They reduce heart attacks in middle aged men with existing heart disease
- They are effective reducers of cholesterol
- They don't reduce heart attacks or mortality in women
- They don't reduce mortality in men who have already suffered a heart attack
- They improve endothelium function
- They have anticlotting effects
- They slow down the rupture of plaque
- They have antiinflammatory effects (Lundell), and reduce CRP levels.

These are actual benefits of statins, which should be weighed up against their many disadvantages and side effects, and the fact that these benefits can also be derived in other ways which do not have the side effects. Besides this, the actual statistical benefits of statins should also be taken into account (see the discussion on the NNT of the statins on p 23).

The cost factor is also of cardinal importance to the heart patient, who is often called upon to consider the following (Lundell):

- Heart bypass: $83 000 (in RSA currently about R300 000)
- Heart catheter with stent: $63 000 (in RSA currently about R200 000)
- Statin medication: $250 per month (in RSA currently about R800 p m).

INFLAMMATION—THE MOST LIKELY CAUSE OF CARDIAC HEART DISEASE

THE STRUCTURE OF THE ARTERIAL WALL

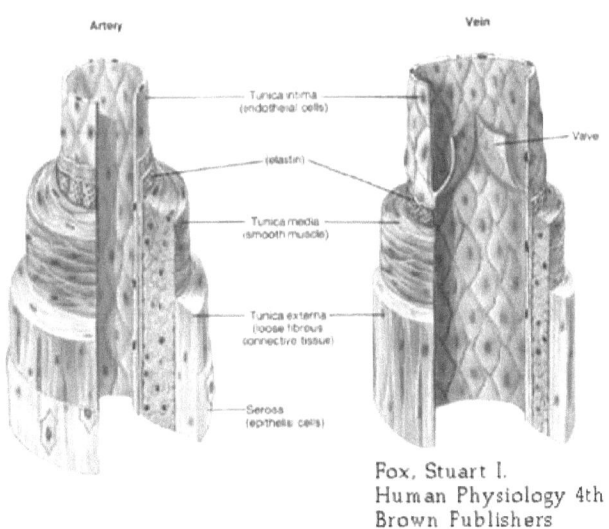

Fox, Stuart I.
Human Physiology 4th
Brown Publishers

Fig. 3

The inner wall of the artery has 3 layers: the Intima, the Media and the Aventitia. This is the case for all types of arteries. There are 6 different types of arteries, depending on the function they perform: elastic arteries, muscular arteries, arterioles, capillaries, venules and venes. The diameter of the arteries decreases in size the further they are situated from the heart, beginning with about 25 mm in the aorta, down to as little as 0.3 mm in some arterioles.

The following are the most important structures of the arterial wall. One needs to have an overview of these in order to understand the process of atherosclerosis.

1. **The Intima** (or inner layer of the wall of the artery): This consists of a single layer of endothelium cells, separated from the rest of the arterial wall by a narrow belt of connective tissue that attaches the endothelium layer to the arterial wall. The Intima is a very thin and sensitive structure and it embodies the direct contact between the blood and the arterial wall. It is probably here that the process of atherosclerosis has its onset, due to inflammatory changes.

2. **The Media:** This is the next layer following on the Intima. The media consists of concentric layers of smooth muscle cells and elastic tissue in a base layer of proteoglycans (carbohydrate molecules attached to proteins) that serve as "cement" material to fill the interspace. These smooth muscle cells make it possible for the arterial wall to expand and contract in tandem with the heart beat whereby the blood pressure is stabilised during the heart beat.

3. **The Adventitia:** This is the outer layer composed of collagen bundles that contain the blood vessels (vasa vasorum). The arterioles offer the greatest resistance to the passage of blood and consequently have a significant influence on blood pressure.

The structure of the Aorta (the first large artery after the left heart) and other large arteries serve partially as blood reservoirs that stretch and contract with each heartbeat. In this manner blood pressure is stabilised.

From the above information (which the nontechnical person need not necessarily learn in detail) it becomes clear that the arterial system is very sensitive and that any changes brought about to its structure (e.g. through damage caused by toxins and inflammation) could have important health implications.

This is the subject of discussion in the following section.

INFLAMMATION

Inflammation is defined as a local tissue reaction caused by irritation, damage, infection or other harmful stimuli such as pathogens, irritants, environmental toxins and damaged cells from elsewhere.

Inflammation is the normal reaction of the body to any attack by which the immune system is activated.

Symptoms will include pain, swelling, reddening of the tissue and, in serious cases, loss of movement or function.

The inflammatory reaction may take place at various levels of intensity, depending on the circumstances. This may include cessation (if the problem has been overcome) or the development of scabs (in more serious cases) when new blood vessels and connective tissue are formed. It may also include the forming of abscesses.

For the ordinary person these are the typical symptoms one observes after insect bites or minor injuries that usually cause acute infections. It is essential to distinguish between acute and chronic inflammation. For the purposes of the current discussion, it is chronic inflammation that is of particular importance.

We usually associate inflammation with arthritis. Inflammation also presents itself as a component of certain chronic illnesses such as heart disease, where it probably plays a far bigger role than formerly believed.

Medical treatment of inflammation, especially of the limbs, includes light exercise, rest, normalisation of body mass (especially in the case of arthritis) and medication. The various drugs that are used to treat inflammatory conditions include nonsteroidal antiinflammatory drugs (NSAID) such as aspirin and ibuprofen, as well as steroidal medication such as cortisone. Initially NSAID are mostly used. These medications are usually well tolerated in the short term but—as with most other medications—they have side effects in the long term, which could include irritation of the stomach and alimentary canal. This could give rise to an ulcer of the stomach or of the small intestine.

An important aspect of chronic infections is the formation of collagen (connective tissue). If an excess of collagen is deposited, a condition known as fibrosis can develop. In this case connective tissue cells known as fibroblasts appear in the area where the tissue has been damaged. They then produce collagen that is needed to replace the tissue that has been lost through prolonged inflammation.

The two most important complications that are caused by inflammation are fibrosis and scab forming. The large amounts of collagen that may develop during chronic inflammation can in time give rise to scab formation, which can cause permanent structural changes to the tissue, and could impede its function.

Chronic inflammation may also be stimulated constantly by processes that have a low antigenic potential, such as certain environmental toxins.

It is most probable that chronic inflammatory processes that form over an extended period and appear on the inner walls of the arteries are the major cause of plaque, atherosclerosis and consequently heart disease.

During open heart operations and also during arterial bypass procedures, these processes can be quite clearly seen at various stages of development in the arterial walls. This is illustrated in the accompanying photographs.

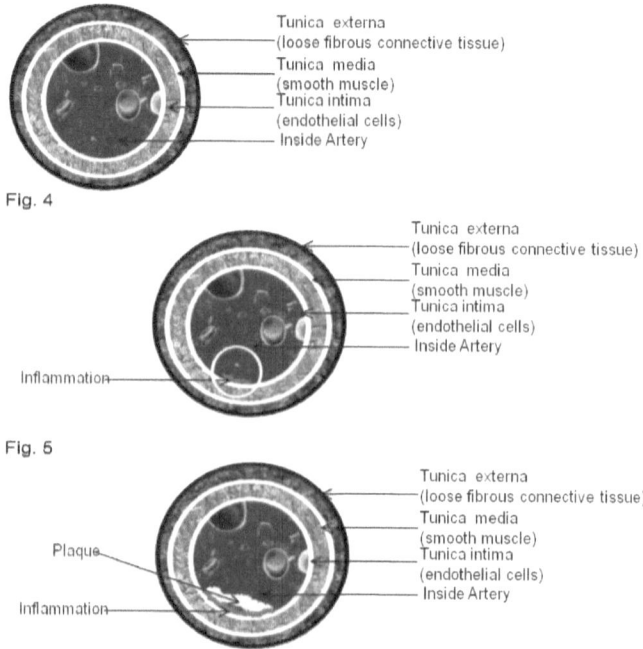

Fig. 4

Tunica externa
(loose fibrous connective tissue)
Tunica media
(smooth muscle)
Tunica intima
(endothelial cells)
Inside Artery

Fig. 5

Inflammation

Tunica externa
(loose fibrous connective tissue)
Tunica media
(smooth muscle)
Tunica intima
(endothelial cells)
Inside Artery

Plaque

Inflammation

Tunica externa
(loose fibrous connective tissue)
Tunica media
(smooth muscle)
Tunica intima
(endothelial cells)
Inside Artery

Fig. 6

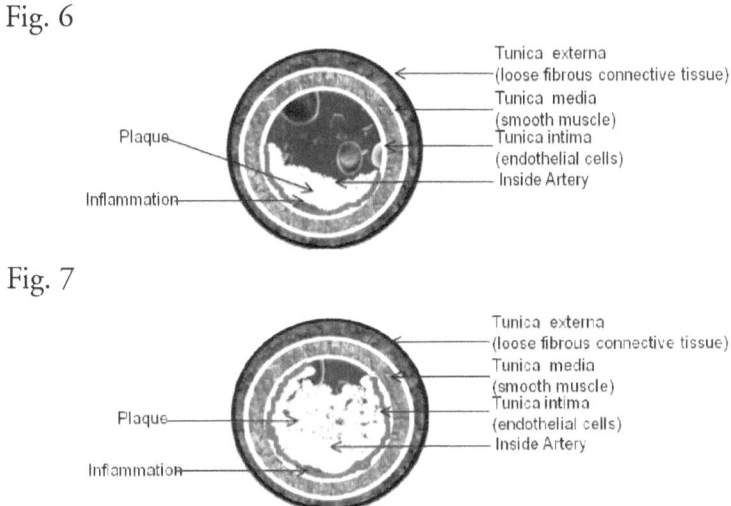

Fig. 7

Dr. D. Lundell, the retired cardiologist referred to above, describes these processes in greater detail in his book *The Great Cholesterol Lie*.

This theory of the cause of atherosclerosis is supported by the composition of plaque and by the fact that rising Creactive protein levels (CRP, a measure of the amount of inflammation in the body) has long been associated with atherosclerosis. This is also reinforced by our own observations concerning the role that stem cells play in coronary lesions, as discussed below.

Further important information concerning inflammation: who is prepared to consider and to recognise these. The areas surrounding coronary arteries where the process of atherosclerosis is developing, resemble an acute injury site where recent damage to tissue has occurred.

- Inflammation is a normal part of our daily existence. It is one of the weapons we have to protect ourselves against infections and other attacks from outside. Widespread low grade inflam mation is to be found in the body following any event that threatens its structure and function, such as muscular pains after heavy exercise, injuries, etc. It is therefore a normal process.
- Inflammation has only recently been recognised as a factor in atherosclerosis, albeit the signsare readily evident to anyone
- Dr Lundell, to whom reference has previously been made, is one of the first researchers to recognise this relationship, and strongly emphasises the connection with heart disease.
- The question immediately arises whether it is advisable to treat the inflammatory processes that lead to atherosclerosis preventatively

at an early stage, rather than to wait until a lesion has developed (perhaps at a lifethreatening level) and then to take action, e.g. by means of heart bypass procedures.

- It is significant to note that inflammatory processes occur constantly all over the body in practically all tissues, not necessarily with harmful consequences, and often without the patient's even being aware of it.

- The immune system is also closely involved in inflammatory reactions. Initially white blood cells (monocytes) are attracted to the damaged area. These cells then send out "messengers" called cytokines for help to ward off the inflammation. This includes substances that cause the narrow blood vessels to dilate in order to carry an increased blood supply to the area (reddening). During this battle some of the monocytes change into macrophages that "devour" dead cells and other debris and thereby remove it.

- Unfortunately not all these processes are as readily observable in the case of inflammation of the cardiac arteries. This is perhaps the reason why it had largely gone unnoticed for so long. This means that we aren't aware of it happening, even though it could have been occurring for years, and could have laid the foundation for what ultimately becomes a heart attack.

CAUSES OF INFLAMMATION

The major causes of inflammation in the artery walls are:

- **Smoking**: Certain chemical substances in sigarette smoke damage the cells of the intima directly, with the result that monocytes and oxidised lipids (LDL) are permitted to penetrate the intima and reach the media. Substances in the smoke also suppress the repair processes in the intima.
- **Blood sugar**: Chronic use of refined sugars gives rise to chronically elevated blood glucose levels, which in their turn lead to chronically high insulin levels. This in turn causes the cells to become insulin insensitive. This is the wellknown metabolic chain reaction which occurs daily in millions of patients in the Western World. What is less well known is that the high blood sugar levels damage the intima layer in the arterial walls, thereby activating inflammatory processes in the artery walls, including all the processes mentioned above. This starts the process of atherosclerosis which ultimately leads to a heart attack. Much has been said and repeated on the damaging effects of smoking, but often the even greater importance of the practical effects of blood sugar is lost from view—many women who do not smoke also have heart attacks. We are not genetically programmed to handle the high intake of refined carbohydrates that are so prevalent in our society.
- **High blood pressure**: The intima is damaged directly as a result of the mechanical effect of pressure, which could give rise to an inflammatory reaction. High blood pressure causes the formation of angiotensin, which is a potent vasoconstrictor, further increasing blood pressure. Reduce salt consumption, normalise body mass, exercise and take fatty acid supplements as discussed here. Should

these measures not have the desired effect, medication can be considered, in consultation with a doctor.

- **Overweight**: Many studies have shown that body fat—especially that around the midriff—is a source of proinflammatory cytochines. In this respect it is true that overweight is both a cause and an effect of inflammatory processes.

- **Shortage of vitamin D**: It is becoming increasingly clear that most of the minerals and vitamins have multiple roles to play.

  This is particularly noticeable in the case of vitamin D. The wellknown role of this vitamin has always been that which it plays in the absorption of minerals—particularly calcium and magnesium—and its role in metabolism, which makes it vital in the formation of bone. New evidence shows, however, that vitamin D receptors are present in many other tissues besides bone, and it has become manifest that these vitamins have a vigorous antiinflammatory effect. This explains *inter alia* why, during the winter months in the northern hemisphere (when there is less sunshine to promote the formation of vitamin D) far more heart attacks occur than during the summer months. Supplementation of this vitamin (2 000 to 5 000 i.u. per day) has become, for this and for other reasons, an imperative in the western world.

- **Lack of essential fatty acids (EFA)**: The EFA is long chain (C18) fatty acids of which there are various types, depending on chemical structure. They are termed "essential" because they cannot be primarily produced in the body but have to be acquired from the diet.

For the purposes of our current discussion there are two types of EFA of importance, i.e. the W3 and W6 families (these names refer to the position of certain double bonds within the molecule and are not of direct interest for the nontechnical person). The three main types of W3 fatty acids are, with the exception of linolenic acid (the mother substance of the family), also the derivatives which are formed in the body from the mother substance, such as EPA and DHA. Both of these are found in fish oil.

The W3 fatty acids are the precursors of the prostaglandin E1 (PGE1) that has antiinflammatory effects, while the W6 fatty acids are precursors of the proinflammatory PGE2.

It is therefore of great importance to maintain a balance between these two types of fatty acids in order to keep inflammatory tendencies under control.

The W3 fatty acids act as nature's regulators of chronic inflammation. They are extremely well suited for this purpose as they have no long term adverse effects on the immune system.

This balance is largely disturbed by the typical Western diet. The correct evaluation of this problem is clouded by two practical considerations, however. On the one hand there is an actual shortage of the W3 series in our diet (e.g. linolenic acid and its derivates) (Lundell, p65). On the other hand there is a false perception that we consume too much of the W6 fatty acids (linoleic acid and its derivatives) because at present our analytical methods do not distinguish between the unadulterated mother W6 fatty acids (linoleic acid) and its derivatives. These are produced when the fatty acid chains in the cholesterol esters are altered during the commercial processing of food sources containing W6, like sunflower oil. We have referred briefly to this problem above (p 20).

In consequence, tissue analysis offers a better gauge for evaluating this matter than the analyses of food products. Regretfully, though, there are conflicting results coming from this at present. On the one hand Prof. Peskin and his associates claim that the W6 series is of far greater importance than the W3 series, in support of which they quote certain substantiating evidence. According to these reports there are far more W6 fatty acids in tissue than W3 fatty acids, e.g. there is on average four times more W6 than W3, while in our skin there is noticeably 1 000 times more W6 than W3 (see e.g. *J Mol Neurosc* 2001, 16:159, 215, and also *Townsend Letter* Aug Sept 2007).

On the other hand, Dr. Lundell points out that, according to known analyses of food products, the ratio is 20:1 in favour of W6, but neglects to take the analytical problems in relation to the oxidation of side chains of cholesterol esters, as mentioned above, into account.

Dr. Lundell further points out that in countries where the tissue levels of W6 are the lowest, the incidence of heart disease is also the lowest (see Lundell, p. 65). He cites Greenland as an example, (W6 level 30) where the incidence of heart attacks was 20 per 100 000, in contrast with the USA where the incidence was 78 per 100 000, with a W6 level of 200. This type of comparison and conclusion is often invalid, however. What other factors in these countries could have contributed to these differences? The actual deficiency of W3 fatty acids in the Western diet could be of far greater significance.

- **Conjugated linolenic acid (CLA)**: Just as in the case of the fatty acids mentioned above, CLA is also not manufactured in the body and must be acquired from the diet (chiefly from meat and dairy products, typically those foods against which we have long since been warned).

Besides its wellknown anticancer effect, further research has revealed its antiinflammatory effect. Furthermore, it reduces body fat, and increases fatless body mass, both in test animals and in people.

Both the size and the number of fat cells are reduced by CLA (Lundell). It is also of particular importance that the CLA reduces abdominal fat deposits, which are now regarded as one of the main risk factors for heart disease, especially in men. The reason abdominal fat is so important is that this type of fat produces more of the cytokines (messengers) which activate the inflammatory processes in the artery walls.

Many cardiologists have reported favourable clinical effects of CLA. One of these maintains that patients who have been treated with CLA lose weight, but that this weight loss is not brought about by the loss of muscular tissue, which is all too often the case with weight reduction programmes.

It also became evident that the levels of Creactive protein (CRP) in these patients quickly decreased to normal levels, which is an indication that CRP suppresses the inflammatory processes.

Further benefits of CLA can be summarised as follows:

- It suppresses the formation of cytochines which stimulate inflammation
- It stimulates the synthesis of antiinflammatory prostaglandins
- It heightens sensitivity to insulin
- It suppresses appetite
- It is a significant antioxidant that assists in limiting tissue damage by free radicals
- Significantly, it suppressed the formation of plaque in test animals by more than 50%

It has become quite clear that CLA supplements are going to play an increasingly important role in the treatment and the prevention of heart diseases in future.

Transfattyacids

Simply avoid all products that contain transfatty acids or hydrogenated vegetable oils, and of course all margarines. The transfatty acids in these products are detrimental to heart patients for various reasons. One such reason is that they compete with the very important W3 fatty acids. The transfatty acids replace the important normal fatty acids in cell membranes and thus disrupt the normal functioning of the membrane, thereby increasing the risk of a heart attack.

Heavymetals

The most important of these are aluminium, mercury, copper, iron and lead. Mercury is of particular importance because the cardiovascular system is especially sensitive to the toxic effects of mercury. The heavy metals as a group increase chronic inflammation through their harmful effect on the production of energy in the mitochondria (the subcellular structures in which energy is produced). They also have numerous other detrimental effects. In one study, the mercury level in the hearts of cardiac patients was found to be 22 000 times higher than in controls. As many of these patients develop cardiomyopathy (lack of energy production in the heart muscle) the conclusion was that mercury in particular acts on the mitochondria, which is the source of energy production. The high concentrations of mercury found in the heart muscles of cardiac patients indicate that mercury tends to collect in the heart muscle. Mercury found in fish from the top of the food chain (e.g. tuna) is an important source of mercury in people. Researchers in Finland found a direct connection beween mercury levels in the hair of parients (which is an indicator of exposure to mercury) and the incidence of heart disease.

A further dangerous source of mercury poisoning is to be found in the mercuryamalgam fillings of teeth that were previously used. The symptoms of mercury poisoning are often to be seen in patients with such fillings. This includes coronary heart disease with no clear cause (absence of the above risk factors) and also inexplicable headaches, confusion, weakness, loss of weight, insomnia, neurological problems, fibromyalgia and fatigue. A more definite diagnosis of mercury poisoning may be obtained by administering an oral dose of dimercapto succinic acid (DMSA) and then collecting urine for the following 24 hours. The mercury level in the urine is then determined and a diagnosis can be reached.

The precise mechanism by which mercury causes heart diseases has not yet been unravelled, but there is no doubt that a connection does exist between them. All heart patients should thus avoid contamination with any heavy metals, and particularly with mercury, by e.g. having mercury fillings in teeth removed by a professional. It is now possible to undergo an intensive detoxification programme by way of chelation therapy, and in sodoing to remove and quantify the levels of heavy metals in the body. See graph, Fig. 9.

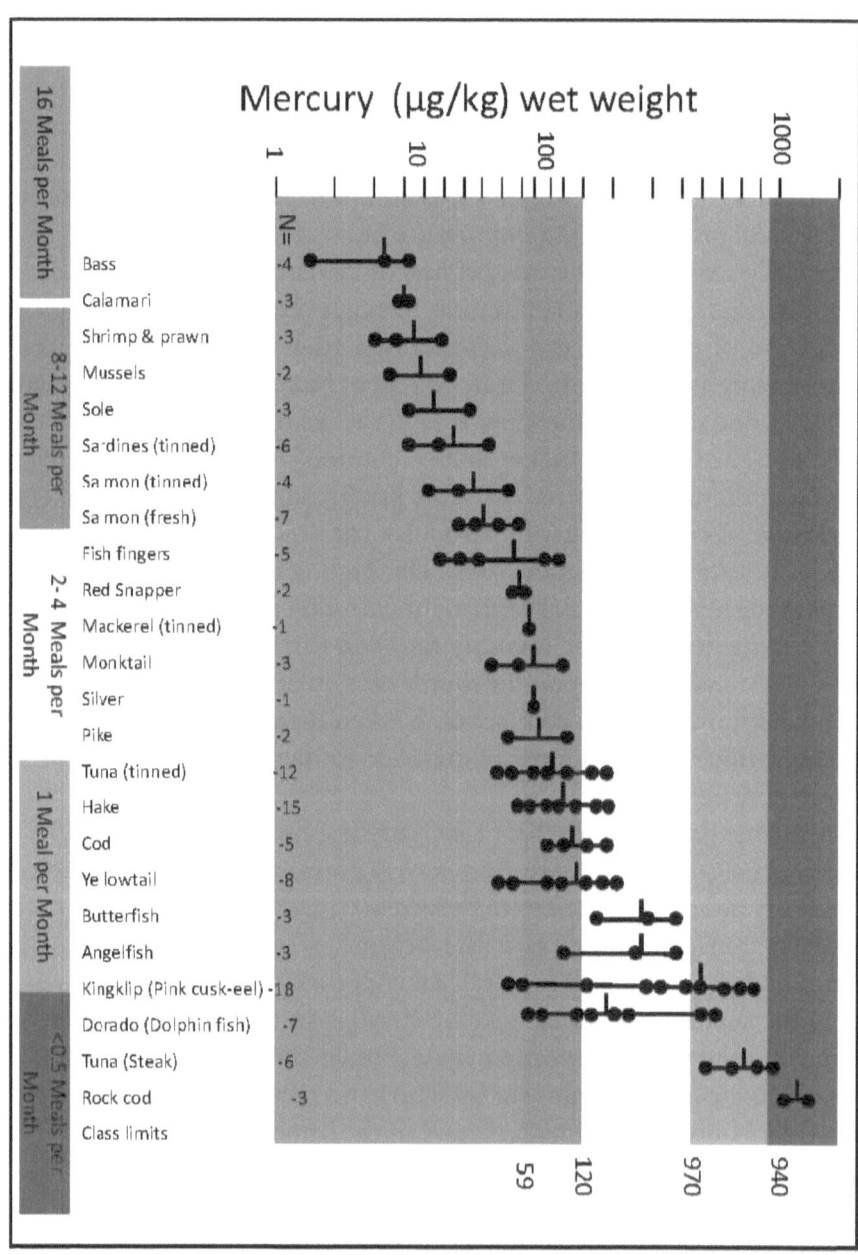

Fig. 9

Freeradicals

Free radicals are unstable, electronically unbalanced molecular fragments, having insufficient electrons. They originate during normal metabolism, and during biological oxidation. Because of their unstable electronic composition, they interfere with many of the body's reactions, including numerous enzymatic reactions, causing metabolic stress. The formation of free radicals in the body is increased by the consumption of alcohol, some drugs, poor diet and radiation. Free radicals increase inflammation and attack cell membranes, affecting cell communication. Besides following the guidelines above, the formation of free radicals can be countered significantly by taking antioxidant supplements such as Vitamins C and E. As cell membranes are largely composed of fatty acids, the fatsoluble antioxidants are of particular importance (alphalipoic acid, Q10 and vitamin E).

Nanobacteriaandothersubcellularorganisms

Although oxidised LDL is one of the factors that initiate the process of atherosclerosis, there are also other factors, some of which have been mentioned above. Besides these, we should also be paying attention to those instances of heart ailments where no clear cause is evident.

Nanobacteria are extremely small microorganisms (as much as one hundredth the size of common microorganisms) and because of this they have mostly been overlooked. They have a significant role to play, however, in those illnesses about which we as yet have little knowledge.

Nanobacteria are probably of particular importance in patients who have heart disease for which no clear cause is evident, and in such cases it is probably wise to treat the patient with a course of tetracycline antibiotics.

Chronicguminfectionandchronicinflammation.

A large number of microorganisms (bacteria, viruses, spirochetes) can be cultivated from the fluids in and around our teeth.

> *There is a significant connection between chronic gum infections and the degree of atherosclerosis.*

This is also evident from the fact that such infections can be associated with increased CRP blood values reflecting inflammatory processes.

It has long since been known that there is a relationship between oral hygiene (gum infections and dental caries) and coronary heart disease. Such infections also bring about lowered immune function.

The most effective method of combating these conditions (besides the usual hygienic measures) is to take supplements that bolster the immune system (Q10, magnesium, antioxidants, essential fatty acids and Immunofood) as well as to undergo a course of tetracycline antibiotics periodically, in consultation with a physician.

Homocysteine(HC)

Oxidised LDL, increased CRP, homocysteine, Lpa, ferritin and fibrinogen are among components of the blood that show the greatest relationship with heart disease. Elevated blood levels of HC are directly toxic to the blood vessels of the heart and brain, and consequently they are a serious risk factor for heart disease.

Patients with elevated HC blood levels (above 14 umol/L) also have a 100% higher risk of developing Altzheimer's disease, and for each 5 umol/L increase in the blood level of HC the risk of Altzheimers increases by 40%.

HC blood levels can be regulated by means of supplements (Vitamin B6, B12, folic acid, and methyl donors such as betain hydrochloride and SAMe.

Many patients (40%) have a genetic defect in their folic acid metabolism concerning the usual folic acid supplements. In these patients supplementing with folic acid will not lower HC blood levels, despite high doses of folic acid and even natural methylators such as betain. These patients should take Metafoline, a highly bioavailable source of methyl tetrahydrofolate that also has the ability to permeate the bloodbrain barrier.

How high should the levels of HC in the blood be? We must first state quite clearly that any level of HC will promote atherosclerosis, but that the rate at which this will take place depends on the levels of HC in the blood. Ideal levels—lower than 7 umol/L—are rare, however. In practice, levels below10 umol/L are acceptable. Levels above 10 are unacceptably high, especially in the case of presenile dementia or when signs of atherosclerotic heart disease are present. Higher levels of HC can be very harmful as it damages the vascular epithelium and increases the attachment of Lpa to fibrin, thereby heightening the tendency of clot formation. In spite of this, one still finds physicians and cardiologists who believe that HC is not important, and consequently find levels as high as14 umol/L acceptable.

Lipoprotein a (Lpa)

Lpa is a blood lipid consisting of LDL that has become attached to Apolipoprotein a (Apo a) by means of a disulphide bond. It is highly proinflammatory and promotes blood clotting. Population studies have indicated that of a total of 5200 patients, those with the highest Lpa levels had a 70% higher risk of heart disease than the rest.

Elevated Lpa levels constitute a serious problem for the clinical cardiologist, because it is difficult to normalise these levels, and particularly because the muchused statin therapy (for cardiac disease) is known to increase Lpa levels. For this reason it is imperative that cardiologists also consider the Lpa levels of patients when they prescribe statins to lower cholesterol levels. It is reassuring to know that the W3 fish oils in combination with high doses of niacin, is often effective in such cases.

Fibrinogen

Fibrinogen is a protein that is synthesised in the liver, and under certain circumstances it can be converted into fibrin to form blood clots. High levels of fibrinogen can be lowered by means of supplements (fish oil, bromelein, green tea, ginger). Excessive levels of fibrinogen are especially prevelant among smokers and postmenopausal women. Levels higher than 3000mg/L are unacceptable. This condition does not manifest in all patients, but if it is present, it must be addressed.

Ferritin Ferritin is one of the forms in which iron is stored, and elevated levels are associated with myocardial infarction (heart disease). The iron in ferritin is present in the form of trivalent iron, which is an oxidant and therefore can convert LDL to form the dangerous oxidised LDL. Such eleveated iron levels may indicate the genetic condition known as haemochromatosis.

Medical treatment for anaemia often entails prescriptions for drugs containing iron, such as salts of iron, or the iron derivatives of organic acids such as iron fumarate, all of which contain nonhaem iron. This type of treatment is often unsuccessful for one of two reasons: firstly, the iron is given without the other cofactors that are needed for the formation of haemoglobin, viz. zinc and copper, and secondly, the fact that nonhaem iron could cause an excess of iron in the blood, which in turn encourages the formation of free radicals and thus increases the danger of heart disease. Those patients, who have low ferritin levels should take supplements containing haem iron together with the cofactors mentioned above. HaemoFood (BloodFood) is an example of such a product.

MEDICAL ANTI-INFLAMMATORY TREATMENT

Aspirin is the traditional remedy for treating inflammation. It is one of the nonsteroidal antiinflammatory drugs (NSAID). Examples are aspirin and Ibuprofen (Motrin). Heart patients must take small quantities (90 mg) of aspirin daily, in consultation with their doctors.

Prednisone is a wellknown steroidal antiinflamatory. It has the disadvantage, however, that it suppresses the body's own synthesis of antiinflammatory compounds in the adrenal glands such as cortisone.

These medications all operate by suppressing the enzyme cyclooxygenase (COX) by which the conversion of arachidonic acid into the proinflammatory PGE2 is retarded.

CONCLUSION

In the absence of more complete information, it would appear that the policy which should deliver the most complete antiinflammatory protection is to take more or less equal quantities of the two fatty acids daily, e.g. 3 g of a high quality fish oil and unadulterated sunflower seed oil. More information on this is available by phoning +27 (0)12 811 0432.

For the prevention of heart attacks, it is preferable to take natural remedies such as the essential fatty acids mentioned above rather than the more powerful but potentially more harmful medications, with the exception of small quantities of aspirin (e.g. 90 mg per day).

THE CONNECTION BETWEEN VASCULAR INFLAMMATIONS AND HEART DISEASE

Healthy arteries have a smooth inner surface (intima) and are elastic, so that blood pressure is kept constant during the various phases of the heartbeat. This changes, however, as a result of inflammatory changes. The arteries slowly harden, and deposits (atheromata) develop, as well as the accumulation of deposits inside the arterial walls. This may eventually cause blood clots, which are the direct cause of heart attacks.

Significant changes take place in the vascular system with advancing age, especially in the intima of the vascular walls. As a result of certain chemical substances that accumulate on the intima, it develops the tendency to attract further deposits from the circulating blood, *inter alia* more monocytes, which further advance the process of inflammation. In this manner the whole process gathers momentum, and eventually the lesions of inflammation develop (scab formation or plaque) which would gradually increase in the average person until a heart attack is inevitable. Plaque that is deposited in the arterial walls can be clearly visible during heart operations.

A heart attack takes place when this plaque ruptures and its contents overflow into the surrounding tissue. The body then attempts to limit its effect by forming a blood clot over the affected area. Such a clot starts forming when blood platelets are trapped in the lesion, followed by the other wellknown sequence of events that lead to the clotting of blood. Clearly cholesterol *per se* is not directly involved here. Should these processes lead to the blockage of a critical blood vessel serving the heart muscle, a heart attack occurs. The constriction of blood supply to a specific area results in the irreversible death of heart muscle, unless the blood supply to that area can be speedily restored.

About 80% of all heart attacks are caused by the rupture of plaque. This is called unstable plaque. A different type of plaque that is not so susceptible to rupturing is known as stable plaque. This can also cause a heart attack, but only if the lesion is so large that it shuts off the blood supply to the heart muscle.

It is important for us to understand that the above events may take many years to develop. It could occur at any time in the average middle aged person's life, however, even in the absence of the usual risk factors such as smoking, obesity, etc. On the other hand, it means that no one will ever have a heart attack out of the blue, without reason. It is a slow, protracted process that affords us plenty of time to do something about it, provided we understand what is going on. The problem remains, however, that the process is very gradual, and there are often no direct signs to trigger our awareness.

> *A further positive aspect is that it is a reversible process which affords us the opportunity to rectify it before it is too late.*

This requires, of course, that we should have methods at our command whereby we can detect the process before it is too late. More about this later.

The formation of scab tissue in the heart muscle means that the muscle loses some of its ability to pump. This may be very slight, so that the patient does not notice it at first, whereas in other cases the patient is clearly conscious of it. If sufficient scab tissue has formed, symptoms akin to congestive heart failure may appear.

The classical symptoms of a heart attack have already been dealt with above.

It is also important to undertand how the W3 fatty acids respond to this process. Firstly, these acids monitor the activities of the monocytes after they have been attracted and attached to the vascular epithelium. The W3 fatty acids prevent overactivity of the monocytes. In other words, they suppress inflammation. There are over 4 500 publications in medical literature that discuss this matter. For our purposes it is sufficient to know that this forms the foundation for the recommendation that all heart patients should take W3 supplements.

CAN STEM CELLS REPAIR A DAMAGED HEART?

For anyone who has had a heart attack, this is a very important question. Those of us who deal with heart patients are asked this question daily, not only because uncertainty abounds in this regard, but also because medical practitioners tend to offer evasive answers to this question.

A stem cell is a cell produced in the bone marrow and has the ability to multiply in any tissue that has suffered damage, and in this way it can become a part of virtually any organ in the body.

There are two types of stem cells: embryonic stem cells and adult stem cells. Embryonic stem cells are those that may be isolated from early embryonic tissue (blastula). These cells have the exceptional ability to multiply *in vitro* (in the laboratory) and thus to become a part of any organ in which they multiply.

Adult stem cells, on the other hand, are found in an organism after birth. Until quite recently it was believed that such adult stem cells can only develop into blood cells, and into the cells of bone and connective tissue. However, in the past few years, it has become evident that adult stem cells have the ability to stimulate growth in any other tissue under appropriate conditions and thus to repair damage to such tissue (*Proc Natl Acad Sc USA*, 94: p 4080).

The current theory concerning stem cells states that they are produced naturally in the bone marrow, and are then transported to all other tissues via the blood stream, thereby becoming a part of the body's natural restorative process. Damaged organs exude "messengers" (proteins) to attract the stem cells to those particular organs. The undifferentiated stem cells in the blood stream then follow the concentration gradient of these "messengers", thereby migrating to the damaged organ, where they multiply and differentiate to become a part of the damaged organ, and consequently a part of the process of repair.

This is a very nice theory, but the problem is that much of the experimental work has thus far been performed on animals, so that information on human stem cells is relatively scarce.

The first cultured human embryonic stem cells were not incubated in a laboratory until 1995. Subsequently, researchers showed that such stem cells could be cultivated for generation after generation, and that they could be stimulated to differentiate to become virtually any cell of the body (heart, liver, bone, etc.) On the other hand, adult stem cells were more difficult to cultivate under laboratory conditions, and could only be made to replicate for a few generations. This led researchers to believe that embryonic stem cells have greater therapeutic potential than adult stem cells.

Lately, however, it has become evident that adult stem cells have the same ability as embryonic stem cells, provided the cultivation is carried out *in vivo* (within the living organism) and not *in vitro* (under laboratory conditions outside of the organism). This indicates that releasing adult stem cells *in vivo* from the bone marrow would produce the same results regarding organ repair as embryonic stem cells.

A further development occurred with the discovery that the rate of stem cell release from the bone marrow into the blood stream could be increased by administering certain chemical substances. One such substance currently available on the market is an extract of a certain fungus (*Aphanizomenon flos aquae*). One of the active components of the extract is known as "Lselectin".

"Lselectin" stimulates the release of stem cells (CD 34+) from the bone marrow.

Another component of such extracts is a fraction rich in polysaccharides, known as Migratose. It is now evident that Migratose guides the movement of stem cells from the blood to the particular organ.

As there are several forms of such extracts available commercially, I shall hereafter refer to this extract as a Selectin Rich Extract (SRE).

Although no extensive clinical experiments concerning the effect of SRE on cardiac patients have as yet been published, case studies that afford hope to such patients have become available. We shall be dealing with one such study in greater detail below.

Meanwhile, certain aspects regarding the practical application of SRE are of immediate significance.

In one double blind study, the release of bone marrow stem cells in human volunteers after administration of SRE was observed. The members of the test group were made to rest for one hour before the first blood samples were taken, in order to establish the base level of stem cells in the blood. The subjects were then divided into two groups: the test group and a control group. The test group were given 1 g (2 capsules) of the SRE, and blood samples of both groups were then taken after 30, 60 and 120 minutes, in order to obtain a quantitative assessment of the circulating stem cells in the samples by means of fluorescence activated cell sorting (FLCS). Next, the experiment was repeated, but the two groups were now switched, to meet the requirements of being truly double blind.

The results showed that the administration of 1 g of the specific SRE resulted in an increase of 25% in circulating stem cells.

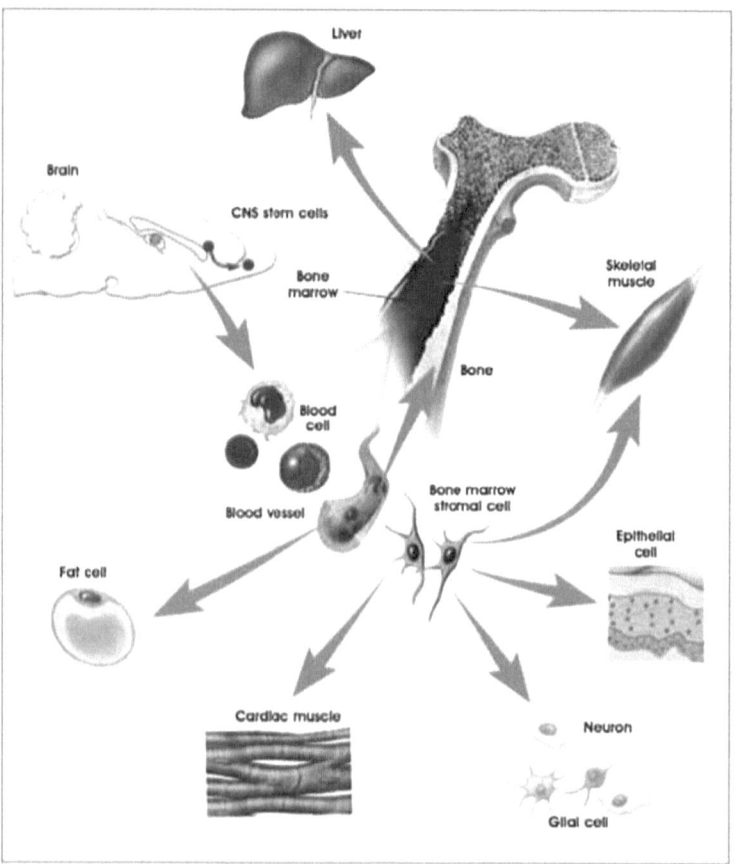

Fig. 10

These findings pose a number of questions, the first of which is whether the supply of stem cells from the bone marrow can become exhausted after prolonged administration of SRE.

This cannot occur, as the body is continually regenerating stem cells at a variable rate. An increase of 25% falls within the normal scope of the physiological variation of stem cells. Such an increase represents some 3 million stem cells, which is a very small percentage of the total number of available stem cells (1.5 trillion). Any surpluses of stem cells not employed for the process of tissue regeneration are simply returned to the bone marrow.

A second question of significance is whether stem cells can cause cancer. There is no evidence that stem cells from the bone marrow can cause cancer.

It has been shown that the extract of Aphanizomenon has antiinflammatory properties, which makes this of particular significance for the current discussion. There is reason to believe that the SRE used for the above experiment has these same properties, although this has not yet been proven.

Besides the effect that SRE has on the availability of stem cells, the increase of stem cells in the blood also offers a number of previously published advantages (*Nature* 9: 1520).

THE USE OF STEM CELLS IN THE TREATMENT OF CARDIAC PATIENTS

There are published studies presently available on this important topic. One such study (*N Eng J Med*, 353: 999) investigated the prognosis of cardiac patients subsequent to the administration of stem cells. Published proof is available to indicate that progenitor endothelium cells promote the repair of damaged arteries (*Circulation* 110: p 2039).

Evidence of beneficial effects has already been documented in a study that indicated that adult stem cells from the bone marrow are able to stimulate the growth of new vascular endothelium cells (*Nat Med* 2001, 7: 439). These experiments were performed on mice subsequent to a heart attack induced by constricting the coronary vessels. This afforded proof that the transplanted stem cells had responded to the "messages" of the damaged heart. After migrating to the damaged tissue, the stem cells differentiated into various subpopulations of cells needed for the repair of the different tissues, including the regeneration of new blood vessels and endothelium tissue.

In further experiments, it became evident that human adult stem cells from the bone marrow are capable of forming vascular endothelium cells. This points to the plasticity that stem cells possess, i.e. that they have the ability to become a wide range of cells differing from themselves, including vascular tissue and cells of the heart muscle.

One possible explanation for this has been put forward by Dr. David Darbro, MD. Whenever specific tissues, such as coronary heart vessels or cerebral cells, have been damaged, as would occur during a heart attack or a cerebral stroke, they send out an emergency call in the form of SDFD (stromal derived factorD) messengers which attract circulating stem cells to that area, where they transform into cells belonging to that particular tissue.

There is a specific system of communication which exists between the stem cells and the cells of the damaged tissue, which provides the stem cells with precise information regarding the exact nature of the damaged cells.

Healthy human bone marrow contains some 150 million stem cells which are gradually released into the circulating blood stream. The exact amount is determined by the health and the age of the particular patient.

At present there are extracts of blue green algae available which have the ability to increase the number of stem cells emanating from the bone marrow. One such extract is being marketed in this country. This product releases some 4 million stem cells daily over and above the normal production rate, after the ingestion of 2 capsules daily. This extract contains a protein known as "selectin", which possesses the ability to stimulate the bone marrow to releases more stem cells. The extract also contains polysaccharides which have the function of enhancing the selectivity and sensitivity of the stem cells, so that they respond even to microamounts of the SDF1 attractors.

A large number of published reports, from a wide range of patients who suffered from a variety of ailments, attest to the benefits derived from taking a stem cell enhancer.

Collectively, these groundbreaking studies have laid the foundation for the application of stem cells for repairing vascular and heart tissue, which now needs to be explored further and on a larger scale in human patients. There are still a number of questions which need to be addressed before these techniques can be applied extensively in cardiac patients, such as:

- How long after damage to heart tissue has taken place will this form of treatment still be effective?
- Can stem cells be specifically programmed to repair only certain types of tissue?
- What type of stem cell are the best—embryonic or adult stem cells?
- Is it preferable to utilise the patient's own stem cells (e.g. from his own bone marrow) or should we rather make use of outside stem cells, e.g. from a stem cell bank?
- Would it be effective to increase the concentration of stem cells in a patient's blood, by releasing stem cells from his bone marrow?

On the other hand, we should bear in mind that no largescale controlled clinical study of stem cell enhancers has as yet been published.

However, the large numbers of positive case reports that have appeared afford encouragement for us to use this product as one of the procedures in the management of postcoronary patients.

The accompanying case study presented below presents us with information that could be the answer to this question. This report concerns a single individual, and as we know, many would reject this type of information as being "anecdotal". On the other hand, there are many who would prefer the results of a single reliable individual above those of a large number of socalled double blind clinical studies that have been "bought" and manipulated by large pharmaceutical companies. In this regard, consider the information presented above on cholesterol, which showed that much information gained from "controlled" clinical studies has had little actual value for the patient—if any at all!

It would thus appear that the normal function of stem cells is to replace tissue that has, through normal processes, become "worn" and/or damaged due to ageing and pathological processes.

REMARKABLE RECOVERY OF A PATIENT AFTER TREATMENT WITH A SUBSTANCE THAT RELEASES STEM CELLS FROM THE BONE MARROW

This patient is a 59 year old white male, Johan. He used to smoke heavily (60 cigarettes a day). At age 51 he had his first heart attack, and it was shown that there was a 75% restriction of the right posterior descending coronary artery. Subsequent angioplasty was unsuccessful, and after 3 weeks the patient was readmitted, at which time a stent was put in position. At this time no further heart damage was observed.

Johan was then put on a strict diet aimed at the lowering of cholesterol, although his total cholesterol was 5.2 mmol/L. The level of LDL cholesterol at the time was 2.8 mmol/L and the HDL cholesterol was 0.6 mmol/L, which is very low. Despite these measures, he had a further four heart attacks 5 years later. He was immediately hospitalised with a blood pressure reading of 230/165, and was stabilised in the Intensive Care Unit. At this time his blood pressure varied widely. Treatment included measurment of heart function, including ECG with appropriate medication. Two days later an angiogram was performed (attached).

The angiogram indicated that the right coronary artery was 100% constricted, and consequently also the right coronary blood supply. A bypass was thus not an option, although a heart replacement was. There was also a restriction of 40% evident in the left coronary arteries.

He was placed on medication, Atenolol 50mg, Prexum Perindopril 4 mg, Elantan Isosorbide5mononitrate 20mg, Simvotin 20mg, Adelat XL 30mg and Disprin 90 mg, en Angised. The patient was then discharged.

While in hospital, Johan heard of a stem cell enhancing product and started taking 6 capsules per day with the approval of the doctors. After 3 weeks he was feeling better, and was able to walk gradually increasing distances before experiencing chest pains.

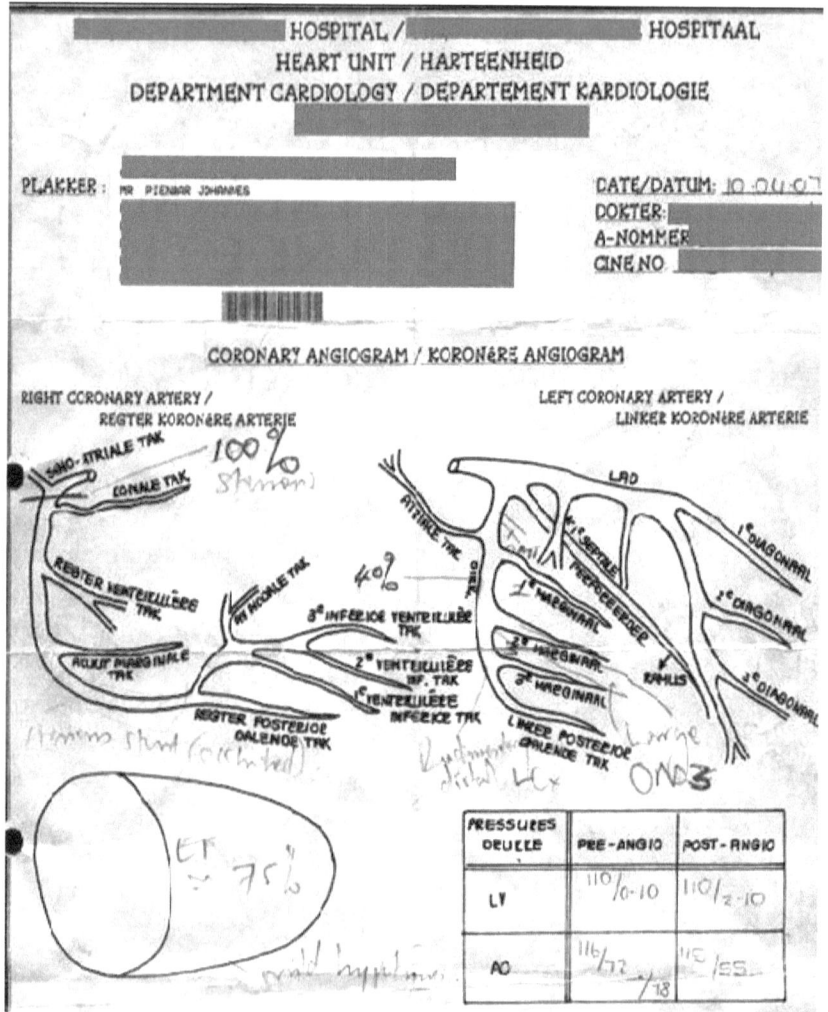

Three months after discharge he returned for a followup visit. By this time he had started to drive on his own again. A repeat ECG was performed, whereupon the cardiologist reported that he had made a remarkable recovery, and should this continue, there was the possibility of a complete recovery.

Four months later the patient was reevaluated, and the finding was that he had made a complete recovery, and he was discharged (7 months after the angiogram was performed).

Subsequently the patient has been returning at 6monthly intervals for followups, and to date he has been stable and no further coronary incidents have been reported. Intensive examinations, including stress ECGs have revealed that the patient has normal heart function. Currently Johan is using no medication, and his blood pressure has stabilised at (average) 126/65.

The exact reason for Johan's dramatic recovery is hard to determine. Three possibilities exist, however:

1. New collateral circulation was established (stimulated by increased stem cells).
2. The increased levels of stem cells in the circulation assisted in limiting the inflammation of the inner artery walls.
3. Increased levels of Vitamin K (also derived from the stem cell enhancer) have increased the elasticity of the artery walls.

More information about the product can be obtained by phoning 082 437 4657

www.ingramcontent.com/pod-product-compliance
Lightning Source LLC
Chambersburg PA
CBHW022128170526
45157CB00004B/1796